NOT YOUR USUAL BOOB

The Good, Bad, and Wonky of Breast Cancer

MK MEREDITH

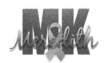

MK Meredith
P.O. Box 1724
Ashburn, VA 20146
Visit my website at www.mkmeredith.com.

Edited by Jessica Snyder
Cover design by Lauren Layne
Cover photograph by Tim Coburn
Logo by Kyung H. Min

ISBN: 978-1-7328980-8-0
Manufactured in the United States of America

PRAISE FOR MK MEREDITH

"Not Your Usual Boob was honest and real, made me think and made me cry. In the end, it made me smile...beautiful and poetic, it has stolen a place in my heart."

— DAWN YACOVETTA

"NYUB is the bosom buddy all patient's & survivors need. When I was going through treatment, MK's insight & guidance would have been everything I didn't know I needed to know. As a survivor, her candor, humor, and honesty makes this the guide we all need to read."

— BESTSELLING AUTHOR HANNAH JAYNE

For every love ever touched by illness.

CHAPTER ONE

YOU

When I got my breast cancer diagnosis, I was immediately inundated with books on cancer. They terrified me.

So, this book...is Not Your Usual Boob.

A little informative, a little sarcastic, a little funny—I hope—and a lot real. This is the book I wish I could have read in my time of need. Some things you can expect during your journey and ways to prepare yourself with a healthy mindset and coping skills before they're needed.

The #NoFilter is exactly that...no filter on the front cover—me and all my wonkiness with no Photoshop—and it's what you'll find inside these pages—including an F-bomb or five. Because more important than shielding myself is being real with you.

You may laugh, you may cry, you may want to punch me in the face...but in the end, remember this. If you ever meet me, I'm hugging you.

Because that's me.

And more than anything, that is the big reason behind this book.

I am still ME.

And YOU are still YOU.

CHAPTER TWO

I Miss You, Mom

I couldn't cry at my mom's funeral.

Two things I don't understand about this. First, I'm a crier. I mean, a huge crier. *Puff the Magic Dragon?* Cried. Hallmark Christmas commercials? Cried. *Tommy Boy?* Cried. And no one cries at *Tommy Boy*!

Don't judge until you've lived a second in my ooey-gooey heart. I'm a feeler, a hugger, and a toucher. If my hands are on you, it's because you matter to me. Touch seems to have a direct connection with my heart. This fact will matter later. You'll see.

The second thing I don't understand about not crying is because I love my mom so much...notice love in the present tense. The feeling has never dimmed. I feel the loss of her every day. So, as you can imagine, my dry eyes wracked me with incredible guilt at the tender age of seven. I couldn't understand what was wrong with me.

Out of sheer desperation and misperceived expectations, I worked hard to produce fake tears to hide my shame. I really believed everyone would think I didn't love her when the truth of the matter was that I loved her so deeply my little brain couldn't accept the reality lying in the coffin in front of me.

I wrote her little notes and stuck them next to her on the satin. I ran my fingers along her cold, firm skin, willing her eyes to open, for it all to be one horrific nightmare.

She really couldn't be gone. But she was.

My aunt scolded me, telling me to keep my hands to myself, and it was one of the rare times my dad rose to the occasion and defended me, saying I could touch my mother if I wanted to. So I did because I couldn't not.

Remember how much touch is connected to my heart?

I couldn't fathom never being held by her or hugging her. I so desperately wanted time to rewind.

I couldn't say goodbye.

But I had to.

And it was devastating. Even as I sit here writing this, my eyes fill with tears as the same feelings from that day wash over me. That's the funny thing about memories, they can produce the same emotion, from anguish to ecstasy, no matter how much time may have passed. Memories are timeless.

I've lived with breast cancer my whole life. At least from my first memories. My mother was diagnosed around the time I was four, waaaay back in the old days just before the early '80's, when the height you achieved with your hair was like an Olympic sport and neon was considered a neutral.

She'd only been 36 years old when she'd received the call, and whether she had been considered old or young hadn't even been on my radar yet. I was only interested in the next time I got to watch Woody Woodpecker and eat donuts. But now I feel the magnitude of her youth with that diagnosis, and at the same time, I feel old with the weight of so many memories and such heartache.

She'd been told over the phone of all things. As the story goes, when she hung up after speaking to the doctor, she picked up an old plaster of Paris bust of Mary—she'd converted to Catholicism after marrying my dad—and threw it against the wall.

I know she felt betrayed.

It landed facing her, upright, without a nick on it.

If you know anything about plaster of Paris, you know this is virtually impossible. And as you can imagine, she immediately calmed.

And found her center.

They told her she had about three months, but she showed the universe. She hadn't been ready, and she lived another three years.

Though she had a mastectomy on one side, and then I believe later the other breast removed as well, the cancer had metastasized to her bone.

Back in the day, you didn't talk about breasts—at least not in public, out in the open amongst respectable people. Not healthy ones and certainly not sick ones. And I don't think anyone had a good grasp on the importance of acting swiftly in the face of cancer.

I'll never know exactly how quickly she sought care or if there had been a better way.

I just know she was stolen from me and my brothers.

And breast cancer was the thief.

She'd been on a medication that basically kept her alive. She and my father decided it was time for her to go off it, but that month, March of '82, my dad's mom died from complications after surgery on her liver. So, my mom went back on the medicine because she wasn't going to have my father bury his mother and his wife in the same month.

Even then, during a time of her own great suffering, she'd thought of someone else.

That generosity of heart was one of her best-loved characteristics.

In April, at 39 years old, with me, the youngest, at 7 and my three brothers at 10, 13, and 17 years old, she passed.

She opened her eyes, said goodbye to our father, and then was gone.

And our lives changed in that moment.

Everything that was, wasn't.

Our family broke.

The reality that had been mine was gone. Though the reality I had was always of my mother being sick, she was one of those special people. You know, the kind you go to visit with the intention of making them feel better but who make you feel better in the end? The part of my life with her in it was filled with such happy memories even though every one of them was made while she was sick.

That's superhero powers right there.

She was my real-life Wonder Woman.

She always gave us time. In and out of the hospital, it didn't matter. She took walks with me and rocked me in her rocking chair while she listened to music by monks from a monastery. She bought that record on a trip we'd taken with my Aunt Kathie to Vermont.

One of the most vivid things I remember from that trip was my mom falling on the sidewalk and breaking her ankle. Bone cancer makes for brittle bones and brittle memories.

I'd been holding her hand, and I've always worried that maybe if I hadn't been, she'd have been able to break her fall without breaking herself. I'd just wanted to be close to her, but with her in and out of the hospital, it was never as much as I wanted.

That night, I desperately wanted to go with her to the emergency room—that yearning sensation is still so very strong—but had to stay with everyone else. Maybe I sensed my ever-shortening time in her presence.

She loved us, loved our dad. She loved being a mother. I don't remember one instance of ever feeling neglected or unloved by her even when she was at her sickest from chemotherapy and radiation. Even the time she gave me a spanking in our car outside of church on a Sunday after I refused to behave. Even then, I remember curling against her side, her silky blue shirt against my cheek, breathing her in, and feeling her love.

I don't remember being told she had breast cancer. It just always was. When she was really sick, we'd visit her in the hospital, and when she was well enough to be home, I'd hang out with her on the hospital bed we put in the master bedroom. We'd painted the walls a bright and cheerful yellow and had yellow daffodil sheets on the bed.

It never occurred to me that she'd die. Even as I sat next to her on the hospital bed. My seven-year-old brain didn't store that possibility.

But the day came when I was called into our family friend's fancy sitting room. It was one that none of the kids were allowed to go into, with velvet-covered couches and fine china vases. I'd been staying with the family while my dad had been at the hospital. My brothers were okay—physically—on their own, but no one wanted them to be responsible for their little sister.

I should have known when I was called into the room and invited to sit down.

I should have known.

The mom took a seat on the edge of the sofa, and I sat on the carpet at her feet. There was no way I'd risk the fancy furniture. I remember the blue of the room all around me. I remember looking up at our friend's face, a halo of light around her head, but not really seeing her as she told me my mom was gone and could never come back.

I remember the devastating clarity of that moment at seven years old, knowing I would not see my mom again. There was no rewind button to push. There was no way to extend the goodbye. I'd never feel the softness of her against my cheek or the safety of her arms around me. Never see her warm smile or feel her hold me. Her voice was gone. Her warm, familiar scent was gone. At seven, my life stretched out before me, and I could think of nothing but how achingly long it would be without her in it.

She was gone. Breast cancer took her.

Stole from her the ability to celebrate life with me like mothers love to do: my high school and college graduation, getting married, having my babies, and publishing my first book.

I know she's always been *here with me*. But it was forever different.

And then it was my turn.

At 39, the year both my little boy, Brody, and my sweet daughter, Anya, had each been 7 at one point or another during those 365 days, knowing their grandmother had died when she had been my age, my husband and I had to tell them...

I had breast cancer.

CHAPTER THREE

Finding the Lump

Christmas of 2014, I walked naked past the mirror in the bedroom of our rented house outside of Washington, D.C. and paused. There was a dip in my breast, similar to the shape you get when you cup your hand. Shallow and wide and due to my long-stored memories and information...menacing. Further investigation with a quick self-exam uncovered a lump.

Some might say I was primed for this moment, but in reality, I was rocked to the core. I'd always watched, always managed my self-exams. I'd even been tested in 2008 for the BRCA 1/2 gene.

I had been negative. LOL! Joke's on me.

Despite losing my mom, that negative test result played a dirty trick on me. It gave me a false sense of security.

And I didn't have time for any of it.

The holidays were here, my favorite time of the year. If I'm not on a beach, I want it to be Christmas. I love the music and the atmosphere. Sure, I see all the commercialization around us, but I also truly believe that every moment, every memory of your life is what you make of it. Sometimes, they are still bad, no matter what we do, but often they can be as beautiful as you want them to be. And I love making Christmas beautiful.

My young children were on Christmas break. The tree and decorations were up. The big day was approaching like the most beautiful summer sun, and there was no way I was doing anything about this stupid lump until after Christmas.

But I knew I needed to act fast.

I made the call, or tried to anyway, the day my kids went back to school.

My husband, Brian, had just taken an early retirement from the Air Force, and it surprised me how many doctor's offices in the National Capital Region didn't accept military insurance benefits.

By the fourth phone call, I broke down crying. At that moment, I had a strong feeling something was very wrong. It wasn't my imagination, and I needed to be seen.

Thank God, the fourth office could help me.

Let me pause to tell you Christmas was as beautiful as I'd hoped it would be. We made memories that our children will take into their adulthood—which is my mission for our lives. Making memories with our family that warm my kiddos when the world doesn't seem so friendly.

I went to my gynecology appointment, hoping I was wrong. At first, in the glaring light of the examination room, the doctor couldn't see anything, so she felt for it. Again nothing. I explained that I personally found it easier to feel when I was lying down. Because believe me, I'd felt for that thing over and over again in the past couple of weeks, hoping each time it would be gone.

Eureka. She could feel something. "Just in case, let's send you for imaging," she'd said.

Yes, let's.

I went for a mammogram. Over twenty-five films later, they couldn't see a thing. My breast was so dense with fibrous tissue that the films looked normal. Had I not been persistent about the lump I felt, they would have sent me home with a clean bill of health. Not because they were incompetent or didn't care, but because diagnostic tools are not perfect, and the films showed what they'd always shown on me.

Nothing.

But because I knew there was something there, they sent me for an ultrasound. Again, "just in case."

And there it was as if I'd asked a toddler to draw a cloud on a rainy day. A round, bumpy, cloud-like image with undefined edges. The tech was new and gasped, so they called for the radiologist.

I hope the radiologist wasn't a poker player, because if he was, he was losing all of his money. "I've seen worse that turned out to be nothing, but just in case, let's send you for a biopsy."

Yes, let's.

I can't think of a single time in my life that the phrase "just in case" has been used as often as it was regarding this lump. And don't get me wrong, I don't find fault with it, but as I'm writing this, the *better safe than sorry* mantra is very strong.

The day came for my biopsy, and my incredibly supportive husband wanted to go with me. Absolutely not. It was nothing, and I wasn't letting him waste a PTO day to sit through a biopsy. Besides, they wouldn't be giving me any results there. I had to wait for those. And at this point, I'd been waiting and waiting and waiting. Or at least that's how it felt with five to seven days between each visit. So, I sent him on his way to work. He argued with me, telling me he knew me better than I knew myself and that he needed to be there.

No, go to work.

I was so, so wrong, and he was so, so right. Damn it.

I'm hoping to keep that kind of statement to a minimum. I am married to him, after all, and need to be able to live with him for the rest of my life without his head growing too large. Ha!

I went in for the biopsy and, while I was waiting, was overcome with emotion. Memories of my mother and her experiences ran rampant through my mind. I thought of my children, of Brian. And I wished that I'd listened and brought him with me.

I was so scared.

But I also had a little guardian angel friend. One of those beautiful and special souls who seems to read your energy from afar, and as I scrolled through Facebook on my phone, trying to distract myself, she messaged me. Just checking in. I don't know if she'll ever understand just how special that moment was for me.

But Rebecca Davis, you, my love, are an angel.

I wasn't alone, after all. She chatted with me until I was called back to the office.

For those of you who haven't had a breast biopsy, my experience was rather benign. The idea of it was disconcerting, but the actual event was very easy, or the practitioners working with me were exceptional. I hope it was a little of both, but I don't want to mislead anyone into thinking it is always easy in case it isn't.

But I can now tell you this. Take your person with you. The one you trust above all others, the one you share your hopes and dreams with. Take them with you. Don't go alone. It can be more emotionally scary than you might first anticipate. And in the end, it's a mere hour or so out of their day. You're worth the time. Do you hear me?

You are worth the time.

I say this because I fall into the same well that so many women, and some men, fall into. That well where everyone else must be lifted up first, where everyone else's needs are to be seen to and satisfied first. It isn't because these other people don't care—it's because we love caring for our loved ones so much that we hate to put them in the position to have to care for us back.

But we're worth it. And so many of them want to do it.

So, don't be selfish—let them care for you.

CHAPTER FOUR

You've Got Cancer

"Yes?" I answered the phone quickly, hoping to silence the ring before waking anyone up. It was the early morning of January 20th, 2015, two days before my 40th birthday, and my brother and his young family were in town to help me celebrate.

"This is Dr. M____."

"Oh, hi!"

"Yes, ummm, hi. I'm really sorry to have to tell you this, but it's cancer."

Just like that.

A funny thing happens to me when I'm uncomfortable. I try to hide it, I try to force the situation to be over as fast as possible. When she said the word cancer, my brain lost all focused thought and filled with a low buzz. Like the white static on an old TV with no connection. Too bad I didn't have any rabbit ears to fidget with.

I heard myself say, "Oh, that's okay. Do you know what stage?"

"The stage and prognosis will be discussed with you at your breast care specialist appointment scheduled for next Friday."

"I'll need to check my calendar," I said.

What? I need to check my calendar? This wasn't an interview or a writer's meeting. This was cancer, but I couldn't break myself out of autopilot.

"Mrs. Meredith, I really think you need to make it work. Again, I'm very sorry."

"Oh, I'm sure it'll be fine." I stretched that damn smile from ear to ear even though there was no one in the room with me to see it. I only had two days left before my birthday.

Two days.

The universe couldn't wait two damn days to let me get past 39? I'd only been waiting all my life.

I numbly disconnected the phone, wanting to run but not knowing where to run to. It's as if you have to act, to do something, yet there is nothing that can be done except wait. It's a cold and hollow feeling. And waiting sucks ass. It does. It might not be nice to hear or say, but it does. I hate waiting with a passion. But I learned quickly, with cancer, there is a lot of waiting.

And I want you to know that, too.

Besides, I couldn't have cancer.

I was a mom. I'd already lost my mom to it. The BRCA 1/2 was negative. I'd paid my dues.

Shit.

I was a mom.

That should be my caveat right there. I had my little boy and my little girl, and they need me. No one else could ever mom them the way I could and would. This wasn't a Disney movie or the backstory of a wounded hero. This was my life.

Panic crawled up my throat, bubbling in my chest, tingling my limbs...then I went numb. I opened my mouth to speak, then closed it, then looked around the empty room, wondering what I was supposed to do next.

I almost laughed, because, come on. This couldn't really be happening.

My heart was breaking.

Then my brother Billy walked in with his usual "What up, douche."—or something else equally brotherly—and dropped into a chair.

"I have breast cancer."

He gave me this look he has that would make anyone else run in fear and opened his arms to me.

I walked over to his chair, fell to my knees, and held on like my life depended on it.

In that moment, I felt like it did.

I was terrified and overcome with a fear of floating away if someone didn't hold on to me tight. He embraced me in a fierce grip, the kind that always left me a tad worried my spine might snap, and muttered something about the Vatican and a massacre.

He was mad.

And scared.

And so was I.

Brian was at work but had told me earlier that he wanted to know, no matter what, as soon as I knew something. Making that call sucked. How do you tell your husband you have cancer? The same kind that took your mother all too soon? While he was at work, no less.

He responded as he always does – with calm, strategic logic. "Okay. We'll see what the doctors say and do what we have to do. You'll beat this."

"Yes, I will."

Always strong, always clear and focused, Brian has grounded me more times than I can count. We both went on with our day, he at work, me at home. I took our daughter to basketball practice, determined that cancer would not touch my life any more than it had to.

It was interesting, sitting there surrounded by a bunch of parents, some with smiles on their faces as they watched their kiddos perform out on the court, some with their noses buried deep into their phones, none of them worrying about whether they'd be there next year to witness another season.

It's weird to have something invisible, something no one can see, threatening your very life. My mind was a hurricane of what ifs and what I wanted to be and the possibility I'd never have the chance. I sat in the bleachers on the constant verge of tears. But that's the funny thing about personal catastrophe. It doesn't matter what—death, divorce, illness—your life just screeches to a jarring halt, but everyone around you continues on in their happy and comfortable existence.

It isn't always easy to see from the outside, and you certainly don't want the people around you to be afflicted, but it might take some purposeful thought to accept and let go of the fact that they are untouched by your tragedy.

And thankfully so.

The fewer people your misfortune can touch, the better. None of us wants tragedy for anyone else, but we don't want to and shouldn't be alone with it either.

So, build your support unit.

Without me realizing it at the time, my support unit grew by one that night because I met a woman at that basketball practice who became a dear friend. Her name is Rebecca. She and her precious family are now our family.

Later, after what seemed to be an endless day, Brian got home from work. He came in with a smile on his face, but I could see the stiff hold of his head, the glassy-eyed look in his gaze. He was pushing through, holding on, and putting on a strong front. He hung up his coat, then went up to change.

I followed him like I always do.

He walked to his dresser, and I asked, "Are you okay?"

Without a word, he turned and threw his arms around me, burying his face in my neck.

My husband—the huge alpha male, logical, physically and emotionally strong, steadfast—cried.

And cried.

"I can't lose you."

"You won't." The thought wouldn't even compute in my own head. It wasn't an allowable outcome.

"I'm scared," he whispered.

"Me, too. But we'll figure it out." It was an overwhelmingly humble experience to have someone so lost by the thought of losing me. I've always known he loved me, but this outpouring almost knocked me off my feet.

I needed to fix this because I couldn't stand the sadness or fear in my hero's eyes.

"You'll beat this," he said.

That was the message I downloaded to my brain as soon as I'd been given the news. I'm a big believer of the body, mind, and spirit connection, so the sooner I could train my brain to think, *I'm healthy and strong and will be just fine*, the better.

I may have gotten the message, "You've got cancer."

But I had a message for cancer.

"You don't stand a fuck's chance in hell."

And with that, I stepped forward.

CHAPTER FIVE

We Have to Tell Our Kids What?!

Wait, we have to do what?

How in the hell do you tell your seven- and eight-year-old children that you have breast cancer, especially when they know your mother died from it?

But we had to.

Brian and I decided we would tell them right away. They are both very intuitive, especially our daughter. No matter how well we tried to hide it, they'd know...they'd overhear something...they'd feel a distur-bance in the force.

The force is strong in this family.

We also know how they work. Our kids don't over-worry about things when they are given all the facts and coinciding solutions. It's when they know something is wrong and don't have any information that they really get scared.

But before we could get to the facts and solutions part of the talk, we had to say the dreaded words.

Brian and I came up with a plan. And I encourage you to do the same.

It may not go exactly as you imagine, but it gives you a solid foundation from which to communicate.

That's a very good start.

We have a wonderful couple in our lives who are our children's adopted grandparents, Kathy and Jim Krans. Kathy is a breast cancer survivor. Once upon a time, we bonded over the learned knowledge that she lost her daughter and I lost my mother on the same day but different years. April 14th was a difficult day for both of us.

It's similarities like this and the coincidences of age and numbers with my own mom that have added layers of interest and unease to this journey.

Kathy had lost her daughter, and I'd lost my mother, and Kathy was a survivor.

It was kismet.

I won't even go in to what brought Kathy and Jim to build a house right across the street from us, but let's just say that we believe her daughter, Veronica, and my mom, Karen, were in cahoots.

So, Brian and I formed a plan where we would lead with the fact that Kathy was a survivor, reminding our kids that many people do survive breast cancer. Then, we would give them the details as we knew them and our plan to wipe it out of me.

We were ready.

Together, we were strong.

On the inside, we were a quivering mess of hearts and guts filled with fear, resenting the fact we had to deliver this news in the first place.

My brother and his family were visiting for my 40th birthday, and their presence was comforting. I know they wanted to melt into the background once they realized what we were about to do, but having them there gave me strength.

And it was important for our kiddos to see they—we—were not alone.

I sat up on the counter so I could have a good view of their faces, ready to guide them emotionally down an accepting and comfort-ingpath.

We led with the encouraging news about Kathy.

And it unraveled immediately.

Our youngest, Brody, immediately burst out, "Are you gonna die?" The sheer terror on his face broke our hearts, and the tears that followed incinerated them. Anya started to cry, too, and I jumped down from the counter, pulling them into my arms. "No, no. You guys. Remember Nana? She survived."

"But your mother didn't."

Well, fuck.

And there it was.

Our kids are smarter than we are. Smarter than our well-meaning and thought-out plans. My mother died. So in their reality, their mother could die. No matter what we said.

On to the facts and our plans.

Kids are amazingly resilient. We told them everything we knew and the plan we were going to take once we got the rest of the details.

They were still scared, but they were so strong.

I told them to ask us anything, to talk to us about anything. No question or comment was inappropriate. Knowledge was power. And I'd happily put it all in their hands.

Off they went to play with their cousins.

And Brian and I sat there stunned.

That was the worst thing we'd ever had to do, and we prayed we'd never have to do anything like it again.

Telling them I had breast cancer was worse than actually having breast cancer.

In the coming months, they took ownership of expressing all of their thoughts and feelings. It was both humbling and heartbreaking when they would get out of the car as I dropped them off at school, and they'd duck their heads back inside. "I hope you don't die, Mom."

I'd grin and throw them a kiss. "I won't."

One night, Anya sat with me at the table, her mind turning and tumbling. She suddenly turned to me. "Mom, what if after you beat the cancer, a month later, it comes back, and you die?"

And Brody, who has always been my snuggle buddy from the moment he was born, came to me with tears in his eyes. "Mom, you can't die. Who would I snuggle with while Anya played video games with Daddy?"

They were the sweetest and most heartrending questions because I knew that no matter how strong they appeared, how well they managed, they were scared.

They were afraid in a way I never was when I was young. In every memory I had at that age, my mom was already sick, and I'd never heard of anyone dying. I don't think her possible death had even been a possibility my brain comprehended before it happened. She'd just been all of a sudden gone.

My kiddos were already familiar with the idea that you could lose people you loved from cancer, and they went from having a healthy mom they never worried about to a mom with something that could hurt her.

And through that, hurt them.

The whole situation made me mad.

And there are going to be times you get mad, too.

Really mad.

Let yourself feel it. Feel the anger. Feel the fear. Feel the overwhelming sensation of helplessness. Roll in it for a second. Validate all of it in that moment.

Then put it in its place.

Feel what you need to feel, but don't stay there. Let it in, and acknowledge it, then set your mind on the path you need it to take to get you out on the other side, alive and well.

For you, for your kids, for your loved ones.

You step forward.

CHAPTER SIX

Screw You, Cancer, I Have Plans

Cancer has incredibly bad timing.

I had the edits of my first published romance due, and Brian had just gotten accepted into an amazing data science cohort.

And I was determined not to let stupid cancer take any of it away.

In the end, I'm glad we pushed through, but it wasn't easy.

I called my publisher, told them what was going on, and made sure they weren't going to change my release date.

Then, I used my writing to not worry about the cancer and dove into the editing process.

It was a bit of a relief to have somewhere else to put my thoughts. A story about a strong woman and a sensitive, handsome man fighting through the ups and downs of life so they can be together, all wrapped with the bow of a happy ending, was just the right place for me.

So, I put my head down and worked away.

My first book came out that summer, my second that fall, and I've never stopped.

You don't have to either.

Don't stop.

I hope you have something that can distract you or help you cope with your diagnosis, that prevents you from dwelling in fear or sadness. A hobby, work, your family, any pleasures that give you a bit of respite will work!

Do these things. Love these things.

During that first week, Brian called me to ask if I thought he should quit the cohort with everything we had going on.

I did not think that at all.

Not *no* but *hell no*.

I knew it would be hard and told him so. I knew it would be stressful for him, but I also knew I did not want him to miss out on such a huge professional opportunity.

If he'd quit, he would have regretted it, and so would I.

In the end, he forged ahead and got through, and the experience has enhanced his performance and abilities in his career.

I'm so glad he called me that day and didn't just decide on his own.

I'm so glad he'd had the fortitude to make it through such a difficult situation at home while taking on such a difficult course load for his cohort.

Cancer, and illness in general, tries to take so much.

Some things will have to go, but so many things don't have to.

Preserve what you can, what is important to you.

Keep living!

Do not put things off, or not do them at all, because you don't know what tomorrow brings. That is the exact reason for you to do all the things!

As you can, for whatever works for you and is important to you, keep grabbing life and running with it. Find your way, keep your goals in sight.

Then, step forward.

CHAPTER SEVEN

Friends, Family, and Fuck Me I'm Scared

Have you ever discovered a spider crawling on you? A big, black jumping spider that looks like it could bench press you with one leg? The sight of it sends a streak of icy cold fear up your spine, and the immediate goal in life is to GET IT OFF. You flick at it, fling it, swipe at it, and smack it, set your house ablaze, and you don't care how crazy you look because leaving Death by Eight Legs on you would be crazier.

That's how it felt to me, knowing there was a tumor in my breast. It was threatening and gross, and internally, I was jumping up and down, swiping at my body like a crazy person, trying to get it out of me. But externally, I had to smile and be patient and...wait.

It's awful. For anyone going through it.

Waiting sucks.

It's a panic you have to live with until you get through the process that begins your treatment, whichever one that may be. It is truly a horrible feeling.

I was like a shook-up pop can. On the outside, I was calm and serene for the people in my life, including myself. But on the inside, I was a bubbling mass of anxiety, fear, and anger.

And impatience.

I had a week before the appointment that would give me details such as the stage, the exact kind, and my probable prognosis. In the meantime, I had to go on with the business of life as I would any other day even though that *thing* was in me.

Your family and friends will be there for you as much as they can be. They will love you and support you, but not everyone knows how, and not everyone is comfortable with their own emotions, much less yours.

I'd been getting ready for my 40th birthday celebration with my amazing sister-in-law. As we applied our makeup and fixed our hair, a bazillion thoughts were racing inside my head. I finally turned toward her and whispered, "I'm scared."

She looked right past me and continued talking as if I'd never spoken. "What time do we have to be there?"

I froze in place, wondering if I should repeat myself—making the situation even more awkward—not sure if she heard me until I really got a good look at her face.

She was scared, too, but couldn't even begin to address it.

Not at that moment.

So, though what I really needed was someone to hug me and validate my feelings with, "I'm scared, too," she needed to move along with the evening and not think about the fact that the sister she loved was sick.

Sometimes, you will need one thing, but the people in your life will need another. I am not in the camp that feels that only the feelings of the one who is sick matters, not when everyone else is affected as well. I want to encourage you to tell the people in your life what you need: I just need a hug, or let me be scared for a minute, or acknowledge my fear.

Sometimes the hug will do the trick, but not everyone will know that unless you say it.

Along the same lines, not everyone will know what to say or how to act, and that isn't anything against them. It is simply a moment where you can express what you need, and you can allow them to express what they need. Not communicating it sets you all up for failure, and not only is that unfair, more importantly, it doesn't lead to success. One of my besties, Kameron, was great at making me communicate. Hopefully you have one of those friends as well.

Everyone acts and feels differently. Some people will hit you with the "everything happens for a reason" mindset; others will tell you that you manifested it yourself—that one feels especially great to hear...*sarcasm*—while others will say, "God won't give you anything you can't handle."

In the end, it isn't everyone else's view on the meaning of life that will explain away why you are dealing with this—it is your own perspective that matters. If you are locked in a negative mindset, I encourage you to do something difficult: Look within, very deep, and find the strength to guide your thoughts. Don't let them run away from you like a crazy herd of wild mustangs, but rather, guide them, one by one, until you have them corralled in a manageable fashion. Your thoughts cause you fear and pain. So come up with different ones.

It makes a difference, I promise.

As I've said before, acknowledge the fear, the despair, the negativity, but don't dwell. Become aware of exactly where you are, the pain you're feeling, and in the quiet that your awareness creates, list all of the things you have to be thankful for.

If you allow negative thoughts to continue to spiral you deeper and deeper, even holding your head up becomes a huge effort. Stopping the downward spiral isn't easy, but when you learn how to do it, it is incredibly powerful.

I cultivated the idea that I would come out of this on top very carefully, but that doesn't mean I was successful all the time. Sometimes, people would say, "Oh, no worries. You'll be just fine," or "Everything happens for a reason." Which I often felt to be true. But there were moments when I wanted to shout, "How the hell do you know?" or "What the fuck reason could that be?!" Sometimes, deep down, I wasn't convinced, and I'd get wrapped up in the "what if I'm not okay" song playing in my head like a broken record.

Those thoughts will come.

And when they do, let them, for a moment. Acknowledge them.

Don't fight it or pretend it isn't there, or it may come back when your guard is down and knock you on your ass. If you see it, really look at it, then let it go. Pull out everything you know about yourself, your situation, and talk your way back up. Because as hard as the journey might be to get back on top, the view is so much more spectacular than when you're drowning at the bottom.

The sun shines, and the birds chirp, and you can look into the faces of those you love and think, *I'm not going anywhere*. You can reenergize your belief that you will get through this, and it will fuel the actual effort you need to put forth to do so. It will fuel your actual body.

Absorb all the love your friends and family offer you. Sometimes they'll say the right thing, and sometimes they won't, but remember they are hurting, too.

Keep all the positivity they pour out within you, and use it to strengthen your own thoughts of health and well-being.

Everything is easier to see with our eyes open—make sure to fill your vision with what you want the future to be.

Then, step forward.

CHAPTER EIGHT

The Cancer of Cancer Books

One of the main reasons I wanted to write this book was because of all the cancer books I was sent home with from the hospital and the doctor's office.

Well-meaning and informative stories filled with facts and figures, and some of the most aggressive language I've ever read. Every one terrified me.

At night, Brian and I would lay in bed, he on his phone connecting with friends on Facebook, and me reading my cancer books. I would sniff, and he'd look over only to discover tears running down my face.

"What's going on? What happened?"

I know I must have looked at him like a wild woman a time or two. "Don't leave me. Should I have gotten more opinions? Did I cause this? Did I, did I, did I?"

"Babe, if the books aren't helping, quit reading them."

Seems so simple, but I'm a voracious reader, and I'm a writer by trade. Not finishing a book is like leaving food on my plate, knowing there are starving children in Africa. I just couldn't. I've forced myself to read books I haven't enjoyed simply because I started them. Silly, I know.

It must have been the third night like this where he finally said, "You need to put every one of those books in recycling. They aren't helping you. They are only making you more scared."

And he was right.

I know many of the books I read will be perfect for many people, but they weren't for me. They were alarming. So this is my warning to you. Some of the books you read will scare you. Many will use language that sends fear through your heart.

And I don't mean the word fuck—you can see I like that word. No, I mean words that should only be used if you're a lumberjack—like cut off and chopped off—not if you're going through a mastectomy.

I went through a double mastectomy and reconstruction.

I knew from the second I was told I had cancer that I would. Back in 2008, when I'd been tested for the BRCA1/2 gene and while Brian and I waited for the results, I'd decided that I would have the mastectomy if I was found to be positive. But I was negative. How ironic.

Christina Applegate was speaking publicly about her ordeal with a breast cancer diagnosis at 36 during this time. When I was researching options and waiting for those genetic results, I came across an article —and I'm kicking myself because I can't remember where the article was from. But in it, the writer described mastectomies like changing the pillow within a pillowcase. We are going in, removing the stuffing that is no longer healthy, and replacing it with some that is.

This resonated with me. This was my voice. It was the perfect way for me to look at the mastectomy. It was a gentle view that allowed me to go through the process and still feel like me in the end. Because that is what I needed.

I didn't want to jump on the bandwagon perspective of losing my identity because my breasts were being changed. The change was for a positive purpose, to keep me alive and well and thriving. So, that is what I focused on.

I also knew that I wouldn't have the mastectomy and not do reconstruction. Some people gravitate to that decision in a natural and beautiful way, and some want to rebuild.

I wanted to rebuild.

So, this pillow analogy suited my personality.

I'm not saying it works for everyone, but I am confident that for those who look at life similarly to me, it is a perspective that can give you peace.

But these books I'd been reading in early 2015 spoke of the whole situation as if it were taking place in a torture chamber. It was shocking. I wish I'd been warned that this was a common theme in many of the cancer books. If I'd known, I'd have never read them.

Then there were the demands that you *must* get twenty second opinions, and that you *must* refuse certain treatments, and that you *must* research to exhaustive measures all the possible treatments worldwide. For some of you, this surplus of information is exactly what you need. But for me, it only added to my fears. It made me second-guess all of my decisions, and it made me question everything I'd learned.

I am a person who needs to gather facts, analyze the options, then make a decision. I don't function well in a life when I bounce back and forth in uncertainty, questioning every second of the day. It freezes me, keeps me from moving forward. This is just me, I realize, but it is also me reminding you that no matter what you're going through, YOU are still YOU.

So use that knowledge. Take it in, and let it settle firmly in your heart.

You need to tackle things in a way that will ensure your success. Don't change your decision-making process because of anyone else, including me. Make your decisions based on what best allows you to process, decide, and move forward. For me, that did not include twenty second opinions.

But I was also very fortunate. The doctors I'd been referred to had wonderful reputations, and what's more, they were exactly what I needed. My breast specialist and plastic surgeon gave me information, options, facts, and supported what I needed to get through this on top.

Find what you need to make your decisions, but don't let yourself swirl in self-doubt because you read in a cancer book that someone else did something different.

That's okay.

Another warning about some of these books is that they may focus on the negative effects breast cancer can have on relationships. I read story after story of husbands leaving wives because their breasts were no longer real. Seriously. Story after story.

I told Brian about it and asked, "We're okay, right?"

He would hug me and tell me again, "Quit reading those books. They're poison."

And they were for me.

Here's the thing. I understand that there are likely relationships that ended for the exact reason the books stated, but to imply that was the most common cause, I feel, is irresponsible. There are so many factors that go into building and nurturing a relationship through all the good in life and the bad.

Factors you need to be aware of so you don't miss seeing what is right in front of you.

For one thing, relationships during an illness will be greatly impacted by the relationship before the illness. Just as in traumatic brain injuries. The prognosis relies heavily on the health of the brain before the accident.

Also, with all the breast augmentation in the world these days, I don't believe that most men can't handle it. In fact, I believe that most men can, that most men are caring and loving and supportive. That isn't to say all are, but you can't say the same for women either.

Another big factor is the person dealing with the illness. A lot of the health of your relationship may come down to *you*. This is the thing. Because we are the ones who are sick, there are those who will say that whatever we are feeling is how we feel. Period.

That is a dangerous and slippery slope. I'm not saying that you shouldn't be strong in your truth. But I am saying that you should avoid—at all costs—using the illness as an excuse to quit being a wife or husband or parent or friend or present.

For example, after a mastectomy, a woman may not feel like a bombshell ready to rock her lover's world. I know I didn't. And I'll get into this more in a later chapter.

Brian and I had a strong physical and sexual connection throughout our marriage. It was something that was just ours, and the more consistent we were sexually, the tighter we were as a couple. So even though I didn't feel sexy as I endured several surgeries to remove the cancer, I tried to find a way to ensure sex remained meaningful and comfortable for both of us. For example, I'd wear a white tank top when we made love. It helped me feel sexy-ish while covering the part of me that I didn't recognize.

I'd hoped it would forge our connection stronger through the treatment process. It allowed me to be held and cherished as a wife, outside of all the times he held and cherished me as his best friend.

Which was beautiful.

But even with this mindset, a few other challenges that I'll discuss later in this book cropped up. I was blind to some very important communication Brian was trying to have with me. At some point during treatment, I got so turned inward by my disassociation with the body I had, symptoms from treatment, and physical and hormonal changes within me, that I missed *seeing* and *hearing* him.

Sure, I put on that tank top and lip gloss, but what he really wanted was to connect. I was trying to give him sex when what he craved was the intimacy we once had. To be seen and needed and wanted as my husband and not just a caretaker. And not as if he was an obligation.

He had real pain, but he never felt he had the right to say anything since I was the one who had cancer.

Your physical and emotional needs should be met, but your spouse has needs and feelings to recognize and acknowledge also.

I had an element of shame, some embarrassment, and a whole lot of denial about what was going on inside of me. I didn't want any of it to be true, and I was afraid I might never get ME back. I have always been a passionate woman, and I didn't want that sexual part of me to be dead, to be gone forever. Though I wasn't feeling like myself, I shoved it down, denied it, and pretended that it wasn't a thing. I ignored Brian's attempts to communicate in favor of rejecting what was happening inside me. I didn't talk to him about it so we could find a new way to navigate.

And it left him feeling unloved, uncared for, and rejected.

That is an enormous regret that will take a while to let go of.

I'd been selfish.

I know this is hard to hear because it is hard to say. But illness is not just about us.

It can't just be about us. Everyone who loves you is affected.

It can also be easy to use the illness as an excuse not to participate in life. Please don't do that. It's hard, I know. Especially if you're going through chemotherapy or radiation. I didn't have to, but I remember all the times my mom did. I don't know how she did it, and I really can't imagine having to, but somehow I never suffered her absence when she went through treatment. I can't imagine how difficult it was for her, but she was always there for us.

It had to be the hardest thing for her to do, but it kept the cancer from stealing away time from us kids, and it kept her relationship with my dad strong.

So, yes, by all means, express what you need. Tell those you love how to help. But give them a voice, too. They are going through this right alongside you. They have desires and fears and considerations that need to be met. It can't just be about the person who is sick, or relationships will crumble. The efforts that were put forth before the illness need to be continued and respected during the illness.

Using the "I'm the one who's sick" route may end on an empty road.

Make sure you get the love and care and compassion you need, but also make sure you are giving it back to those who make up your life.

Communicate the truth. Don't get stubborn or selfish or closed off.

And be careful what you read. Make sure it strengthens you and offers direction instead of weakening you with fear and indecision.

Then, step forward.

CHAPTER NINE

Opinions are Like Assholes

For real.

It doesn't matter what you have going on in your life. Naming your child, which college you should attend, to breastfeed or not to breastfeed.

Everyone has a friggin' opinion.

And before you mistakenly think your own opinion matters, everyone is always right, too.

Even when you have breast cancer.

Let's back up a bit. Once I had the final diagnosis, I posted about it on Facebook.

I'm a romance writer. People know me for high heels, peanut butter, and hugs. I am pretty much an open book and find that I cope with things much better when I can be forthright and honest about them.

So I shared my news on Facebook with all of my readers, followers, and friends.

· · ·

Hey there my lovely friends. I am beyond humbled to have received such amazing birthday messages, and I hope to respond to each and every one. I appreciate your friendship and well wishes for my turning 40!!

I have a little bit of news to share, and for those who know my brothers and I lost our mom when she was 39 from breast cancer, it is kind of a slap in the face...but my stupid boob got the cancer. I have stage 1 as of right now. So, a small area on the left side. Next week we'll figure out if it spread, which could make it stage 2. I plan on getting a double mastectomy and reconstruction, I will be on a lovely cancer med for the next 10 years, and chemo will depend on what we find out next week. Fingers crossed that I don't need it because I really like my hair.

LOL!

I will be fine! I have an amazing husband and kiddos, brothers, and all of you.

Stupid boob cancer doesn't stand a chance. I wanted to let you know because I'm not a bottle it up kind of gal. Big surprise, right?

Hugs and squeezes to all of you!

And no sad faces...they're just sad. LOL!

The outpouring of love and encouragement was overwhelming. I couldn't keep up with all the care and good thoughts sent my way. Brian and kiddos would go on to my page and read what people posted because they were comforted by the love, too. Never in a million years had I expected people to respond like that.

To this day, I'm blown away.

What doesn't always feel great is that your openness (and everything inherent to social media) invites everyone else's opinion as well. I did my research; I made my decisions. That isn't to say I'll never go back and consider a change or put myself on a new course, but by my 40th birthday, I was very comfortable with who I was, what I knew, and what needed to happen to give me the best chance to see my kids graduate and say, "I do."

I caught my cancer early, which significantly improved my prognosis, but I also accepted that there were chances it could come back.

I got a double mastectomy and reconstruction and was put on Tamoxifen for the next ten years. My cancer was hormone receptor-positive, so the Tamoxifen's job is to fill the hormone receptors on any existing cancer cells—if there are any—to keep them from triggering or growing. My mom was diagnosed at 36 years old and died at 39, and her mother also had breast cancer, so I am supposed to be on the medication for ten years.

And boy, oh boy, there were plenty of people who wholeheartedly disagreed with my decision. I received messages telling me to reconsider the poison I was putting into my body, to quit all medicines and simply go on a strict vegan diet, even messages telling me I should or should not get the mastectomy. It was crazy.

Well-meaning, no doubt. But crazy.

So many people putting their *shoulds* on me. And it wasn't helpful.

These messages left an itch under my collar. One I had to deal with because I'm the one who put my situation out there for the world to see. However, it was the right decision for me, because over the following year, I was held up consistently by all the love and encouragement I received.

What a beautiful and excruciating surprise. By opening up, others began to reach out to me with questions or a need to talk. Helping them also helped me.

Yes, I continued to get "You should" messages, and I'd just leave them where they were.

This is a warning for you that everyone will have an opinion on what you should be doing, but it is up to *you* to do what is right for *you*.

For me, dying was a real possibility even in the twenty-first century. I had already lost friends and continue to do so, and I'd lost my mom. Having children who were the age I'd been made me sensitive to any risk. There was a bigger risk in not taking the hormone blocker than taking it, in my opinion. And the mastectomy and reconstruction were absolutely necessary. There was no way in hell I could live, not knowing what was going on in my other breast.

Not with how fibrous my tissue was, not after twenty-five films from the mammogram showed nothing days before an ultrasound detected my cancer immediately.

No way.

I know me, and when you're going through any kind of challenge in life, knowing yourself is vital. It doesn't mean you never step out of the box or leave your comfort zone or avoid all risk. It simply means you know at your core what you can and can't live without.

I knew I'd live in fear every second of every day if I didn't do the double mastectomy.

I also knew I could not *live* that way.

So, my decision was made. I'm also very fortunate to be married to my best friend, who discussed everything with me and who, in the end, was comfortable with whatever I needed to do.

My mother's story was never far from my thoughts, either. After a mastectomy, her cancer came back in the other side, then spread to her bones. The idea that my cancer could be anything like hers made Tamoxifen the right decision for me.

On top of surgery and medication, I was exercising every day, taking vitamins and supplements, increasing my vegetable and green tea intake, and working on losing the extra weight I'd put on over the previous year. All of these things have been shown to decrease recurrence, but I was taking the medicine, too.

My decision went totally against the opinions of some well-meaning friends, and that's okay. Everyone will want to share their knowledge with you, not because they're Bossy McBossy Pants, but because they care about you and want to help.

Each of us have lived a uniquely individual experience that colors our perceptions—it affects the foundation from which we see the world, and it's demonstrated in the opinions of everyone in your life. But they are not you. Don't let their suggestions make you afraid or angry or frustrated. Accept that they are offering you hope. Keep what helps and what works, and release what doesn't. But above all, don't let it freeze you into a place of indecision.

Everyone will have an opinion, but the most important opinion is the one you can LIVE with.

Go, figure out what works for you.
Then, step forward.

CHAPTER TEN

Mirror, Mirror, on the Wall...You Bitch

Apparently, I was so disconnected from my breasts immediately following my mastectomy that I was offering to show them in mixed company. Inappropriate company, like our good friends, including the husband—and their daughter. It's embarrassing to admit now, but it's what happened.

My openness wasn't meant to be creepy but rather an "It's so weird to me; it must be weird to you, too...wanna see?" kind of way. There were moments when I'd felt a bit like a circus show under the big tent. Granted, I was on some heavy medications, coming off of a lot of anesthesia, and just generally muddled physically and emotionally from what I'd been through.

But my husband and best girlfriend, Paula—who came to stay with us a few days helped keep me in check. LOL!

I'll be honest. I really embraced that pillowcase analogy when it came to my mastectomy, but there were times when the need to meddle with my breasts at all wore at my positivity. I've learned that

I'm really talented at pushing difficult thoughts and situations to the back of my mind and simply ignoring them. Not processing each and every detail. I get to it eventually—usually—but sometimes, I need to compartmentalize the when and how into much smaller units and then visit them once I'm ready. Bit by bit.

Immediately following the mastectomy was one of those times that I temporarily shoved any thought that wasn't in line with my positive pillowcase analogy to the background until I could get a better hold on things.

Because the fact of the matter was, I was still me, but there were things I'd read, things I'd seen, and a few of my own thoughts that were trying to challenge that fact.

But it was true. I was still me through and through. Regardless of the change to my breasts, that would work itself out anyway. In fact, I was *more* than still me—I was a stronger me. Hell, I'd been handed a breast cancer diagnosis, scheduled my mastectomy within the month, and was on the road to recovery.

I didn't hesitate. Action was what gave me peace because I am a person who doesn't do well with pain. Which isn't necessarily a good characteristic.

You may need something different. The point is to know what that need is. And to embrace it. Let it carry through each step that you take. Only you really know what those steps are. Your doctors will make recommendations, and well-meaning friends will have suggestions. But you have to decide what is right for you and your family.

And then, do that and continue moving forward.

During this process, be warned...

Your mirror image may try to set you back.

Don't let her. She's like the mean girl who knows you're amazing and tries to knock you down to make herself feel better.

You will look in the mirror, and you'll see your face, your shoulders, your hands, but your chest after a mastectomy—at first—may look a bit like a deflated beach ball covered with stitches and tape.

It's better to know this now, so when you see the beginnings of your new breasts, you're prepared and can think...*All right, I know you. You'll get better. You're what gets me to the next step.*

Then you continue to move forward until you're feeling whole once again.

When you do move...literally, take it slow.

I was sent home after the mastectomy with a three-day pain pump (epidural-style) in my back.

Thank God.

Because the very first time I sat up and the tissue expanders shifted against the just evacuated tissue inside my chest, it was like sandpaper against a burn. I could manage it, so don't worry...you can, too. I just wasn't expecting it. And holy hell, was I really happy for that pain block. I can't imagine how that would have felt without it.

The block gave my body three days to heal, and the pain eased up before I was facing each movement with regular pain medication alone.

When I woke up from my mastectomy performed by my talented breast care specialist, Dr. Elizabeth, I was presented with a pink basket from an incredible organization called the IIIB's Foundation. The basket was a collection of items that other survivors had found helped in the recovery process. Travel pillows to support your arms, tea for an upset stomach, a mug, lip balm, warm socks, a blanket, and a back scratcher. There was more, but these are a few of the items that really brought me comfort.

It was a symbol that I was not alone. Many women before me had been through the same, and unfortunately, many women will go through the same after me as well. But the basket from the lovely women at IIIB's Foundation was a sweet light, a wish for a speedy recovery, an understanding of what was lost and what was gained.

I enjoyed every well-thought-out item. Later, they added a lanyard that could be worn around the neck to support your surgical drains while you bathed.

Now bathing was an adventure! LOL! Brian had to help me at first. No one warned me that my range of motion would be so limited.

I found out after the fact that during surgery, a good amount of your chest and front (anterior) shoulder muscles are actually held out of the way while they clean and check your armpit (axillary) area.

For me, all of this manipulation made my muscles clamp down afterward.

Plus, my chest muscles had been cut to make a pocket for my tissue expander and implants. So, I could barely lift my arms a few inches. Let me be clear—it wasn't that I was in excruciating pain that couldn't be handled. My doctors had a smart and proven plan to help me there. It hurt, sure, but my pain was managed. My body simply limited the range of motion in my arms.

For someone who had been lifting at the gym a week before, I had a hard time handling this.

I just want you to know so you aren't taken by surprise, so you aren't scared that it will never get better. It takes time, and you have to be patient with yourself—which can be extremely difficult to do—but you will regain your range of motion.

I was stubborn and didn't go to physical therapy. I used to be an occupational therapist and was determined to be my own patient. I diligently worked through wall-ladders in the shower—place your fingers on the wall at waist level and finger-walk your way up as far as you can each day.

Once cleared, I also took my ass to the gym and worked through range of motion exercises with a stick.

That was quite a scene.

One day, I got so frustrated with my inability to lift my arms all the way above my head that I started to cry.

And couldn't stop.

Good lord, woman. Get a hold of yourself.

I hid my face, pretending to look for something in my gym bag until I could get myself under control, but I'll never forget the feeling of helplessness and the hopeless idea that I'd never fully recover.

Just so you know...I did.

And you will, too.

Save yourself the frustration, and go to physical therapy if it's recommended. I would have obtained greater range faster and with less heartache with the right help. My stubbornness was not beneficial.

Now, back to the surgical drains. Let someone help you. They are gross if you aren't used to seeing that kind of thing, but in the end, it's just tissue and fluid, not poison. We all really need to get over ourselves with these weird limiting perceptions of our body and its functions. Have someone help you. It'll make it a lot easier.

Drains can be itchy or feel a little like a bee sting if tugged or moved the wrong way, but they are an irritation more than anything else. Getting all the extra fluid out will help your insides heal much faster and keep your pain lower. So, acknowledge the PITA they are, and then be thankful.

All these different challenges you notice in the mirror, from the visual aesthetic you wake up with to the limits of your body and drains and tubes, are all things you can handle. Knowledge is power. Knowledge allows us to plan and prepare.

You're on your way back to you.

Look in the mirror.

Smile.

Then, step forward.

CHAPTER ELEVEN

Triggers and Guilt

I was always surprised by what triggered me during my recovery. I think the timeline for when this happens and the triggers themselves will be different for everyone.

It's kind of like when you lose a pet, and you're used to them following you around. You get up, make your coffee, lean against the counter to take your first sip, when you realize the little furry shadow that at this point is usually nudging your leg for attention...is gone.

And you are suddenly swamped with the feelings of loss all over again.

Triggers were kind of like that for me.

But they weren't always a reminder of what I perceived I lost due to my cancer. Sometimes fear was triggered, sometimes anger, and sometimes pity. I ran the gamut of emotions on a daily basis.

I was busy writing, forgetting for a moment that cancer had ever touched my life, when my daughter walked in and asked me to take her bra shopping. The sudden awareness that she had boobs and I could have somehow passed this genetic bullet down to her filled my heart with fear and stole my breath.

The guilt of having anything to do with something that might hurt her in the future was more painful than the mastectomy.

Another time, I was surfing through Facebook, and I came across a video of a woman finishing chemo. It showed how the nursing staff surrounded her with love and adoration. And in a flash, I was crying and sad, hating that anyone had to go through such fear or treatments that had to hurt while they helped. A race to the finish line, fingers crossed that the victor was the help and not the hurt.

Memes, posts, messages, posters, ribbons.

Breast cancer seemed to be more everywhere than ever before. And I bet it feels similar to those forging their way through other cancers out there as well.

Once you have it, you end up meeting so many others who have survived or are going through the same. You'll also hear so many stories about those who didn't make it. Those stories are a persistent reminder of your mortality that, frankly, I could do without.

But you will hear these stories, and you may meet other patients who are not doing well, who may not be well.

It is scary, and for some, it can lead to a bit of survivor's guilt.

Know that this can happen, and have someone you can talk to about issues like this when they pop up. Don't be like me and be too stubborn to go...that stubbornness did not serve me well at all.

There is no rhyme or reason behind those who make it and those who don't outside of the physiology of the disease itself, actions taken, not taken, timing...luck. That part sucks.

I prefer science and things that make sense. But illness doesn't always fit into a neat little box like I'd prefer.

In situations like these, I find myself feeling guilty that I get to be okay. I get to hold my sweet little boy when he's scared and comfort my daughter when she's upset, look into my husband's eyes each morning when we wake up.

How was I so lucky?

Which is funny because I certainly didn't feel lucky when I was diagnosed.

And this brings me to my main point.

Your thoughts and emotions will be all over the place. Perspective and context make a huge difference in the direction our thoughts and emotions take. Ride with it, but have action plans to help make the journey as smooth as possible. Be honest with your feelings; then think about all the things you are grateful for to help avoid spiraling down a negative path.

You may also encounter guilt when dealing with other family members or friends who are fighting cancer but have to live with it for the rest of their lives.

There is no cure for cancer, only treatments that range from successful to not. Other people may thrive despite the diagnosis but may not necessarily consider themselves survivors because they'll live with cancer until they can't anymore.

The emotions around this disease are myriad, and you might sway from feeling guilty—*why am I the lucky one who gets to be okay?*—to indignation when someone talks to you like what you have been through wasn't hard or scary simply because now you *are* going to be okay.

Or you may be the patient whose cancer has spread, and you will be treated for the rest of your life. On the flip side, you might feel resentment toward those who get to live cancer-free.

All of these feelings are very real and valid. It is important to acknowledge our own reality, to accept our weaknesses, and celebrate our strengths. And you might be in a position where you don't know yet where your path leads, where your journey is going to take you.

It is often helpful to identify ahead of time what steps you'll take for any eventuality. Determine ahead of time who you can talk to, who you trust for the right information, who can help you be strong when you feel weak, make you smile when you are sad, calm you down when a hatred you don't even recognize boils through your veins.

A trustworthy support system will be one of your greatest tools for handling your illness in a healthy manner. Having more than one person to talk to will help prevent you from overwhelming those you love, because if they love you back, they are going through some version of this, too.

Yes, in a different way, but it is still affecting their lives, causing them fear, and producing change, and it is important we remember that, too.

Then, step forward.

CHAPTER TWELVE

Pick Your Poison

I hate to say it, but as you wade through the treatment options, you will see that a lot of it is kind of scary. No, scratch that—it's not kind of scary—a lot of it is just plain terrifying. Because it seems like in order to fight this damn disease, we have to risk other injury or awful side effects.

Science has made tremendous strides, and I read about new possibilities all the time. Possibilities that seem to isolate the cancer cells and may be more gentle on the body. If you are able to consider procedures like that, I think they're definitely worth research.

I, however, am definitely triggered by the loss of my mom, the fear of dying on my children, and the uncertainty of time. So, I wanted to hit and to hit hard. I knew years before my diagnosis that I would have a mastectomy—a double mastectomy—due to the fear of the BRCA 1/2 gene I was tested for in 2008.

After extensive research and deep discussion with Brian, I decided that I would get a mastectomy prophylactically if my test results were positive. But the universe is a sneaky bitch.

I was negative.

Now, don't get me wrong. I am so thankful that I was negative because that lessens my chance of cervical cancer. But the negative result certainly gave me a false sense of security, making me a bit more surprised than I should have been when I did get my *you have cancer* call.

The decision to have the mastectomy had already been made, so I told my physician right away that I wanted to schedule my surgery.

They performed an Oncotype test, which tells the doctor the benefit-to-risk ratio for chemotherapy, helping more than it would harm or harming more than it would help.

My Oncotype was low, and chemo was not recommended.

I was so relieved.

Unfortunately, I have many friends who have life-long residual effects from the chemo. I am telling you this because I will not lie to you. I will also tell you that if my Oncotype was anywhere within the range telling me that I should do chemo, I would have been first in line.

I will not mess around when it comes to my children.

I don't doubt that there are potentially more natural and healthier ways to treat cancer than the Oncology Gold Standard, but until those are proven and backed by science and accessible in a way that makes treatment fast, I have to stick with what feels most comfortable to me.

One of the things that frightened me while reading a lot of the cancer books were all the recommendations to get second opinion after second opinion after second opinion. Or the opposite end of the spectrum where the recommendation was to refuse poisonous Western medicine and to heal only through a plant-based diet.

It went from one extreme to the next. I'm not saying that any of the suggestions are wrong or that they don't work, but for my state of mind, it wasn't helpful.

I really liked my doctors, and if I didn't, then I would have changed, no question. But because I was comfortable with them, because they took time with me, and they answered all my questions... they gained my trust.

I was confident in their experience and abilities, so I was able to find comfort in their treatment suggestions that complemented my own research and find a way to move forward. I'm not a person who can wait and plan and plan and wait.

I had to take action.

You may need something totally different than what I did, and that is okay. Figure out what makes the most sense to you. Identify what brings you the most comfort and peace. Take in as much of the advice that resonates with you as you can handle, and ignore what you don't want because, in the end, you have to be at peace with the decisions that are made.

There is another thing I will warn you about, and that is your wonderful, loving, well-meaning friends. Some may criticize your choices because of something they read or events they've gone through or things they've seen. I do not think that there is any maliciousness to this at all. I truly believe it comes from a wonderful place of love and the desire to see you well. However, it is not always helpful.

I did not want to continue hearing other people's voices in my head, trying to make me second-guess what was right for me. Obviously, if you hear something that makes sense, then look into it, but don't automatically assume that someone else's decision or choice is more right for you than your own.

If you are in a position to do some research, to fly to specific centers that are performing world renown cancer innovation...then do that, and share the information with the rest of us.

I started off with Pick Your Poison, but what I really mean is choose and own your voice.

Then, step forward.

CHAPTER THIRTEEN

Trying to Be Me

There is something very elemental about seeing your body as *different* than it used to be, regardless of the catalyst—pregnancy, weight gain, treatment from an illness.

However, when you don't have control over that catalyst, I think it hits harder and in a distinct way because you don't have to simply get used to the new visual you...

You have to accept and move past why you look different.

When you survive an illness, some people won't understand what difficulty you possibly could have because, hell, you're alive, aren't you?

If only it were that easy.

Yes, you did survive, and you gained an understanding, a perspective that provides gratitude and relief that you are still here. But gratitude and frustration are not mutually exclusive, so it's not always easy to shut down other emotions like resentment that you have to live with these physical changes you never asked for in the first place.

My bra size used to be a 36G. That is way more boob than anybody needs. LOL!

My chest had a funny life cycle because it—I—bloomed way late in college. I jumped from a B to a double D then back down to a B then up and then down again...my hormones have always been all over the place.

Due to those drastic changes—and no, my weight didn't change at the time, only my chest—by around the age of 24, I felt like my breasts had settled into somewhat deflated balloons. So I got implants to lift those suckers up and feel better about how I looked naked. I was so happy with the results I ended up being a 36DD, what I considered the perfect size for me at 5'9" with an athletic build.

Well, those crazy-ass hormones of mine kicked in when I had my children, and my boobs grew and grew to the point that when I breast-fed, one boob was way bigger than the head of my baby!

It was a pretty freaking funny sight to behold. And those boobs are the ones I ended up getting used to because I had them the longest. I had cleavage in a turtleneck. And they were an important aspect of my sexual relationship with my husband.

After my mastectomy and reconstruction, I was a 36DD again, back where I had been before having children. The size looked nice, and I know that they weren't small, but because I was so big before, it was quite a mental adjustment.

I would look down and think, *oh, look at my little baby boobies!* They appeared so small to me but seemed big to everyone else. And my clothes fit differently, too. I would try tops on and take them off and try them on and take them off, and nothing seemed to fit well.

At least, not how clothes used to.

One of the harshest physical changes came thanks to the Tamoxifen I was prescribed.

I gained thirty pounds in three months.

Outside of pregnancy, it was the first time I'd ever put on weight like this. I never had the freshman fifteen, never gained after getting married. I lost the weight after my children.

But on Tamoxifen, nothing I did stopped the damn pounds from finding a home...mostly on my belly.

So, on top of having smaller boobs, my waist and thighs were much thicker. Honestly, most people didn't really notice—a few friends who pay closer attention could tell I'd gained a little bit, but to them, it didn't seem like a huge change.

I couldn't recognize myself.

Here I was, just turned 40 with smaller boobs and a bigger gut (see the cover photo). My clothes didn't fit. I didn't feel well, and it just fucking sucked.

Can I say that? It *fucking* sucked.

I know—I was lucky to be okay, to be alive, and I recognize that someone in a different situation might say, *I wish I had the problem of smaller boobs and a bigger gut.*

But for each of us, whatever moment we are living in, that is our struggle and our reality, and I am telling you right now that your feelings are yours. They are valid and not to be dismissed.

That doesn't mean we roll into a ball and tuck our heads away from the world and quit living. It simply means that it sucks, and now we have to figure out the steps to get back to who we are.

Time helps. Taking action helps. So make a plan, and see what works for you. As far as my breasts go, I just had to give myself time to recognize my reflection as me. To look at that person in the mirror and give her credit for where she was and how well she was really doing—how damn perky those boobs were.

I'm going to let you know this, too. Once you get through reconstruction, your worst critic is going to be yourself. You will notice any little thing that is out of place, any asymmetric characteristic from one breast to the other. So be gentle with yourself, and give yourself time to accept the person you see in the mirror as well. To accept her and be kind to her—or him.

My weight has continued to be a struggle. I've always had to watch what I eat, and I've always had to exercise. That did not change. In fact, I exercised more consistently and harder during this recovery than ever before, yet I was not seeing or feeling any changes in my body.

I tried Atkins, a modified low-carb Keto diet, intermittent fasting, and calorie counting. The weight would not go away. I didn't gain more, but my body would not release a pound. It never went into fat-burning mode. It would only use what I was eating and break down muscle for glycogen, so I never got any gains from lifting weights either.

But thank God, I kept doing it, or I would have lost a lot more muscle than I did.

It drove me crazy when doctors tried to tell me it wasn't the Tamoxifen or that breast cancer patients become more sedentary, or my favorite…"You just turned forty, so your metabolism changed." Just like that. *Snap!* Here's an extra 30 pounds nearly overnight. I don't think so.

I understand that your metabolism changes, but it does not just switch off the day you turn forty. There are chemicals and hormones and all sorts of interactions within our bodies that make that happen. And those responses from doctors are dismissive and lazy and can drive you batty.

I love the advances Western medicine has made in oncology, but with some things, breast cancer patients in particular, doctors get lazy when they don't know how to help you find a solution. So just know that if you're eating well and you are exercising and you're still gaining weight, I feel very strongly that it's your medication.

Doesn't mean you stop taking it. It just means you know the root cause.

Depending on the medication you are on, you may have to learn to manage the side effects because being on the medication is more important than being thin. But don't let dismissive opinions make you feel like you've failed. Ask for help. Consult with a nutritionist or dietician. Research options. All of our bodies are different.

The weight gain had moved me up two pants sizes. My blazers and tailored shirts would not button. I couldn't wear anything fitted because I looked like I was four months pregnant, and my feet were swollen.

It was frustrating as hell, and it made me even more mad at the cancer.

I finally found a solution, but it included changing my medication and a combination of other things, all of which I will explain later. Just know that we are all individuals, and we each have to research and explore what works best for our particular bodies. If you know you have a sensitivity to medications, then talk to your doctor early about ways to handle side effects, both physically and emotionally.

The emotional part is what will floor you. It is what will steal moments from you. It is what will screw up your memories. As I said earlier, I should have joined a support group and started to see an oncology therapist, and I highly recommend that you do. Don't be stubborn like me. It only causes you, and maybe those who love you, unnecessary pain.

I also want you to ease up on yourself, and know that in time, you will figure it out. That you are worthy and strong and a dynamic person who deserves to feel good about yourself.

Do you hear me? Repeat it. Out loud.

I am worthy and strong and deserve to feel good.

Then, step forward.

CHAPTER FOURTEEN

You Don't Have Cancer Anymore, But...

For those of us fortunate enough to be pronounced cancer-free, it may be the beginning of your struggle with gratitude and apprehension.

At least that's how it was for me. I was so relieved that my body was free and clear, but at the same time, I couldn't shake a constant sense of fear. Now that I'd had cancer once, every pinch, pain, burn, cough, hiccup, breathless moment, and numbness in my body set off an adrenaline surge of fear.

What if it spread? What if it was coming back? What if there was something wrong, but the doctors don't see it?

We all hear about the advantages of catching cancer early and the challenges involved when finding cancer late. It can be helpful to have strategies in place for any potential situation that you may face.

Let me be clear. I'm not talking about thinking worst-case scenario where you worry yourself sick with what ifs. Worrying about the future or being sad about the past is not a productive or rich way to appreciate your present.

I've learned that the hard way.

But having a plan to deal with something difficult helps lasso your thoughts and yank them under control so that you can move forward in a healthy way and not spiral into negativity.

I strongly believe in the mind-body-spirit connection.

The power of positive thinking is real. That doesn't mean that we neglect or ignore the negative thoughts—it means we implement a plan to face them head-on and don't let them dictate where we are going. Because remember: You are strong and worthy and deserve to feel good.

I don't think the fear that something else could be going on ever really goes away, but you definitely can manage your relationship with that fear.

You acknowledge it. You accept it is there. You let yourself feel it for a second. But then you focus on reality, whatever it is in that very moment, and you pull that into focus to help you realize you are breathing, your heart is beating, you are well, and you are capable.

If you notice something different, you go to the doctor and get it checked because you have learned to be proactive and to be your own advocate. You have choices and options. You are not at the mercy of your fear—instead, you will use that protective instinct to be stronger and healthier than ever before.

There is also a weird, I don't know, disconnect or something about the idea that you are a cancer survivor, but you no longer have cancer —compared to a cancer thriver who is doing well but may have the disease for the rest of their life.

You had cancer, but you don't anymore. So where do you fit? Do you fit with everyone else around you who has never had cancer? Are you only a survivor? Should you sit with the thrivers?

I don't know that we need to sit anywhere as much as we need to be really present in each moment and be aware of who we learn from the most. From talking to cancer thrivers, I've learned that they really need to connect with other thrivers, other warriors dealing with having cancer that may be reined in but not eradicated, because a survivor won't understand.

People who live with a long-term cancer diagnosis are at a stage in life that survivors never reach. They no longer have the same challenges and have different levels of fear. In some ways, they may even feel a little resentment toward a survivor—not because they wish anything bad on others, but because they wish something different for themselves.

As a survivor, we need to find those who help us the most. Another survivor, your best friend, your mom...someone who can be available no matter how many times they may have already heard the same story. To really process big things takes time and repetition.

Find someone who understands the symptoms and side effects you're going to be dealing with. You are cancer-free, but there are still challenges. Speaking with someone who has already dealt with side effects and symptoms and the fear of it coming back, or someone who can help you work through options and process your feelings may be life-changing.

And even when you do find a great person, or people, or a group to talk to, I still highly recommend you talk to a professional. Issues that you don't recognize or anticipate can sneak up and make your life harder than it needs to be.

So, acknowledge your fears, feel them, face them, then set your path toward healing.

Then, step forward.

CHAPTER FIFTEEN

Where do I Belong, and How the Hell Do I Manage This?

How in the hell do I manage this?

This was a big question for me when I was assigned to an oncologist. I was super excited because she was a professional woman my age, so I was thrilled to be treated by someone who would relate to my issues as a woman, as a mother, and as a professional, both physically and emotionally. Unfortunately, that was not the case.

Tamoxifen causes different reactions in different people. Some people may not have a negative experience at all while others will endure so many side effects that the medication is changed or they go off it altogether against medical advice.

My side effects were horrible, and it became my new normal to the point where I didn't realize how bad I actually felt until I stopped taking it. More on that later in this book.

While on Tamoxifen, I gained over thirty pounds in under two months, no matter what diet and exercise regimens I followed. I had achy joints. I still fought with acne due to hormonal imbalance. Not sleeping was the regular. My mood fluctuated, and I had an overall feeling of malaise, almost like morning sickness. I was fuzzy-headed and fatigued, which made focusing and working out that much harder. I also had terrible water retention—a few hours on my feet, and my ankles swelled to be as thick as my calves.

I went to this new doctor armed with questions and excited to get some answers.

My cancer was hormone-positive, so I couldn't take medication that would affect my hormones or increase my estrogen. And I was interested in natural and effective remedies as well.

At my first appointment, I asked my oncologist about the water retention. She said she would not put me on a diuretic and that she didn't know about any natural remedies that could help. When I asked her about the weight gain, she said it wasn't from the Tamoxifen and that she didn't care how much I weighed as long as I was healthy. So on and so forth, with each question, she dismissed every side effect I asked for help with, telling me to just be healthy.

I started to cry from utter frustration. She stood and gave me the most awkward half-pat hug, told me she was sorry that I was "having a hard time with this," and then she walked out of the room.

I get it. Her focus is making sure I don't have cancer anymore, but my focus is having a life that I want to live. My focus is not feeling like shit every day. Not losing myself.

I struggled to hold on to who I was.

I felt like I was dropped in the ocean without a life preserver and expected to find my way back to shore on my own.

I needed help with my water retention, carpal tunnel, acne, weight gain, cloudy head, and everything else, and her answer to me was to just "be healthy."

Yeah, that's what the hell I was trying to do.

But I'm not a doctor.

What I am is a strong and determined woman who will stand up and be an advocate for myself at every turn.

And you must do the same.

I found a new oncologist immediately.

The doctors I have had in all the other areas of my cancer treatment have been outstanding. My breast care specialist, my plastic surgeon, my radiologist, and the new oncologist...all wonderful. They listen to me, they hear me, and they help.

One of the things you deserve and must demand, if necessary, is a doctor who will listen with both ears...with respect. No one knows your body as well as you do. And this will come up later in the book as well. So stay tuned.

So how did I change doctors?

My breast care specialist has a team member called a patient liaison, Laura, and she is a miracle and an angel and a gift. She knows who she is, and I hope that if she ever reads this, she accepts how truly significant and powerful having her there for me has been through all of this. She was a huge part of me fighting to find my voice, my comfort, myself.

And from the bottom of my heart, I thank her.

The patient liaison is someone you can turn to with questions, concerns, and complaints. I went to her right away after my unfortunate visit with the first oncologist and sent her a five-page dissertation on how unhelpful the doctor was to me.

This sweet angel read my concerns and addressed each one, taking them seriously, then helped me find another doctor. She encouraged me to find someone who worked for me and my personality needs. Find the specialists who fit you.

Because you know what?

That oncologist who wasn't right for me may have been and will be the perfect fit for somebody else.

Some people are more comfortable with a doctor who focuses on the science of the disease rather than the emotions of the patient. Others appreciate a softer bedside manner from their practitioner. Neither is right or wrong, just personal preference.

I changed doctors and found a sweet man who listened with his whole heart, mind, and spirit. He was right up my alley with a nurturing demeanor and encouraging words. Even though he was a man, he understood my frustration and my fears, and we worked through options to find a solution for each one. We looked at science and statistics, and he shared his knowledge.

He didn't just want me to survive. He didn't just want me to be healthy. He wanted me to be happy and to love myself as well.

So, don't be lazy. Be your greatest advocate and find the doctor who provides what YOU need.

Maybe it is the direct and cool physician or maybe it's someone who wants to discuss your emotional health. Only you can determine what the right fit is. But really pay attention to what is in your heart, what gives you comfort and strength, and then find those characteristics in your doctor because you are going to be visiting them and trusting them with your care for years to come.

Cancer isn't over just because you don't have it anymore.

Your doctors will continue to see you and suggest lifestyle changes to help make sure that sucker stays gone.

To ensure I'm not just as guilty as the physicians of not offering up any helpful solutions on managing symptoms, in the back of this book, you'll find a short list of some of my side effects and what helped me. But remember, I am not a doctor, so they are only descriptions and based on my personal experience. Always talk to your doctor before you make a change to your medication, diet or exercise program.

My cancer is gone, and I have a treatment plan for the next ten years. A huge benefit for me was dodging chemotherapy and radiation. A not so huge success is that I don't feel great on Tamoxifen and the side effects that come along with it, but I know I have so much to be grateful for, and I'm no quitter.

I'm working out five days a week, I jog, I do yoga, and I lift weights. I'm not seeing huge results physically in the mirror, but I am getting stronger. And the trick is to keep going.

So now it's figuring out how to thrive as a survivor and make this my best life.

Then, step forward.

CHAPTER SIXTEEN

What Do You Mean It's Back?!

What the fuck.

A little over two years after my first diagnosis and double mastectomy, I was watching *Lucifer* with Brian. Love that show! Tom Ellis makes an amazing Lucifer Morningstar. My husband loves him, too. LOL!

Anyway, we were watching Lucifer, and Brian was giving me back tickles. It's one of the things we do when watching a show. It's a nice way to spend time together and unwind and feels amazing!

I had an itch on my breast and felt a little bump. It was right around the areola, and I'd had nipple-sparing surgery, so I automatically assumed that it was just a suture or a little bit of scar tissue. But between my mom's history and my own experience, there was no way I was taking any chances. I called my plastic surgeon the next day.

She took a look and also thought it was most likely scar tissue but, just in case, she removed it right there in the office for testing. I walked the sample to the pathology office across the street to expedite the process.

I was in the midst of starting a new job after staying home for eight years with my children and writing full-time. It was a period of huge mental and emotional transition, not only for me but our kids, too. We were also buying a new house, which is a mind-boggling experience with the cost of living in the DC Metro area. We moved into an apartment for about five months until our home was finished.

The logistics of starting a new job, moving, changing the kids' school and generally getting into the swing of things was a lot to manage at one time.

The call came on Friday. I was due to start work on Monday. I was sitting at a Starbucks, having just dropped our children off at school, and decided to give myself a little last day of freedom treat when my phone rang.

It was my plastic surgeon, and I had every expectation that she was going to say, "You're in the clear," but instead, she said, "I can't believe it, but it's back. I'm shocked, but it's back."

And once again, I was left in a state of numb surprise. How in the hell was it back?

Ahhhh, hello, this was not convenient. I was just about to start a new job. I didn't have time to do all the appointments again.

But even more overwhelming than the stress of appointments and the unknown was the immediate sense of feeling hunted. That statement probably sounds dramatic, but I'd had a full mastectomy. I had clean margins with the thinnest skin flaps my surgeon had ever seen. I stayed on Tamoxifen. I was doing everything I was supposed to do.

Why did it come back?

I've talked to doctors who say all it takes is one cell and recurrence is easy, but I've talked to others—like my breast cancer specialist—who say that I was the poster child for a breast cancer patient who should be a twenty- or thirty-year survivor and is shocked to see that the cancer came back.

My breast cancer specialist said she'd presented my case at a conference because the combination of my profile, thin skin flaps, and clear margins made everyone believe I was clear.

It was the same kind of cancer as before, so it is was considered a recurrence versus a metastasis or a new type...which was very good in a lot of ways.

So, I pulled up my big girl panties. I'd done this before—it wasn't new—I could do it again.

And that's just it. There is no I *can* do it again; there is simply I *will* do it again.

I had to. My diagnosis was treatable, doable, and not as bad as many of my friends. Inconvenience, fear, and exhaustion are not good excuses to quit.

Besides, all the inspiration I ever needed was always right in front of me.

My children.

They are so strong. They were already frightened once, and I hated the idea of having to scare them again. I was pissed and apprehensive, but I was here.

And I planned to keep it that way any way I could.

If this happens to you, you can do the same.

Then, step forward.

CHAPTER SEVENTEEN

Appointments and Breakdowns

The next week was a bit crazy.

The first thing I had to do was tell my brand-new employer, and that didn't go over very well. They responded that of course my health was the most important thing, but if it disrupted the job more than a few days, I would have to seriously consider whether or not this was the right position for me.

Basically, it was, "Hey, we hope you're fine, but don't let this cancer affect your work. Don't let your cancer affect us."

I don't think they meant to be callous. I just think they didn't consider what they were saying before they said it.

I swiftly went from being pretty excited about the job to feeling pretty offended. I get it—in business you want to make money. But personally, the moment we put the value of a dollar higher than the value of the person standing before us, we've made a mistake.

I started my training with that passive-aggressive warning in the back of my mind. Then, all the phone calls for my myriad doctor appointments started pouring in. I got the call from my oncologist immediately and ignored it at first. Not because I wasn't facing my diagnosis—and no, I wasn't putting myself in danger by not addressing the new tumors. I didn't ignore it that long—but I knew the oncologist wouldn't really become active in my treatment until after the surgery that would remove the cancer.

My first week of my second breast cancer diagnosis was spent in training, so phone calls and appointments had to be fit in at the end of the workday or scheduled for the following week. And believe me, when you have cancer in you, you want it out—yesterday.

I hated that I had to juggle any of it.

I hated that it had the nerve to come back. Son of a bitch.

It was stressful, but juggle I did.

When you are diagnosed with an illness like cancer, there are various appointments. I have an amazing breast care specialist who did my mastectomy and followed up every six months. I have a plastic surgeon I adore, and there's my sweet oncologist.

As much as I love these people, I don't want to see them all the time. LOL!

Since my cancer is hormone-positive and it reoccurred, my consultation list also included a gynecologist to talk about my ovaries and a radiologist because I wasn't going to get out of this one scot-free.

The Tamoxifen apparently hadn't been able to block the amount of estrogen I made—a cell was triggered and started to grow. The first suggestion in the treatment plan was to go off the Tamoxifen.

Thank. God.

Congratulations to me! I hated how I felt on that medicine. Weirdly, I never realized exactly how awful I felt until I was able to stop taking it. The relief was swift and significant.

Next, we'd do surgery to cut out the cancer in the breast, and they would shut down my ovaries with a shot called Lupron. I would have to stay on the Lupron for ten years, and it came with a whole new slew of side effects.

Hell. No.

Been there, done that, no way.

So, I did my research.

I was already forty-two. The idea of having to inject myself or get injected with a medication for a decade that would make me feel like crap was as unappealing as regurgitated vomit.

I spoke to some friends who had had their ovaries removed and were on Aromasin. Losing your ovaries in your early forties has consequences—low to no estrogen can have effects on heart health and bone density...not to mention you're thrown into immediate post-menopause.

But I knew that for my situation, especially considering how crazy my hormones had already been, the best thing I could do for my body was to give it a break. I told my doctor I did not want to do the shots; I wanted my ovaries to be removed.

She asked me a few questions because she really wanted me to consider all the consequences of my choice. The possible good and the possible bad. When you are a hormone-positive breast cancer survivor, you can't or shouldn't supplement with hormones. This meant that however my body responded would be what I was left with. For some people, it is awful, but for others, it's the right procedure.

I considered everything carefully, but I know my body. I'd been fighting my crazy hormones for years, and this was the moment I needed to be an advocate for myself. This was the moment I felt I knew what I needed more than anyone. Now, I understand that can be a dangerous frame of mind, so I caution all of you to discuss options honestly with your doctors, do your research, ask your questions, and then determine your best course of action.

In this situation, I put my foot down and shared with her that after my experience with Tamoxifen and all the side effects and forums I'd read on Lupron, the shot was a hard NO.

I wanted my ovaries out. Luckily for me, she agreed it was our best bet as well due to my history. But she warned me about the effects of being slammed into menopause. After the way I'd been feeling for the past two years, I was willing to take that risk. Personally, I think one of the reasons menopause is so hard is because your body is in flux, hormones unbalanced, for a long period of time. People may not realize how much a shift in hormones impacts how you feel, your energy, your sleep, your ability to focus, and so much more.

Menopause sucks for most women. That's why we all hear all the jokes about it and why there are so many stereotypes about women going through it.

I felt like doing it slowly or taking the Lupron would be a helluva lot worse than just taking the ovaries. So, we scheduled the surgery.

Once again, I found my cancer early. I count myself very lucky. It had not spread to my lymph nodes. Though I did have to have radiation on the left side, I did not have to have chemo.

Science over emotion was my answer.

Medically, early detection and localized cancer cells meant I did not have to do chemo, but then my oncologist threw a wrench in our conversation and told me that if emotionally I felt like I needed chemo in order to make sure that the cancer didn't come back that we could do it.

What?!

On one hand, there is a part of me that enjoys taking charge of my treatment. On the other, the doctor is the expert, and I want to know what they think.

Many of my friends who've had cancer have gone through chemotherapy. I remember my mom going to her treatments. She was such a trooper. She would come home feeling sick. She lost her hair, and the medications caused swelling, but she kept me from ever feeling bad about her treatments. She always loved, hugged, held, and spent time with us. I thought about her a lot while trying to figure out my own path. She was never very far away.

I told my doctor, "Science." I was—*am*—terrified of cancer returning again, but I was more afraid of the potential lifelong side effects or damage from chemo if my treatment plan didn't warrant it.

Let me make this clear...if I'd been told the chemotherapy was the best answer to helping ensure the cancer did not come back, I would have done it. I will do whatever is necessary to be here for my children. The loss of my own mother is way too fresh for me to screw around—even after thirty-seven years. But that's me. You have to know you.

Finally, we had my treatment plan in place. Surgery to remove the cancer in my breast as well as taking out my ovaries. I'd switch from

Tamoxifen to Aromasin now that I was post-menopausal. And I'd have radiation on the left side.

Radiation was five days a week for a month and a half. I scheduled it at 7:00 a.m., before my workday began, to make sure that *it didn't affect my job*. In addition to those daily appointments were the continual checkups, pre- and post-surgery appointments with my breast care specialist and the OBGYN, then the surgery, and follow-up appointments with my oncologist.

I'll be honest with you.

As emotionally well-balanced as I think I am, there were more than a few days where the stress of not letting my cancer affect my job got the best of me. I would feel so angry. So angry that I would go home and talk with Brian and spiral out a bit and break down in tears.

He would give me his ear and would listen, and then he would snap me out and pull me back up to my feet again. I'm lucky because that man understands me. He understands that I need to acknowledge and really feel my feelings, and then I need to let them go. I am not someone who can say "I'll be fine" without acknowledging that I'm scared as fuck first.

Prepare yourself for many appointments. Think of ways you might be able to mediate the intrusive and disruptive pain in the ass that appointments can be. Scheduling, making some back-to-back, figuring out transportation and day care. Let your friends and family help. They'll want to but might not know how. When they say, "What can I do to help?" Tell them. Don't say "Nothing, I'm good."

Appointments are there to make sure your team can give you the best care possible, so having a positive mindset about the necessity of them will help.

Hang in there, and be gentle with yourself.

Then, step forward.

CHAPTER EIGHTEEN

Self-pity and Fear Make Awful Bedfellows

I read a line similar to the title of this chapter in *Eat, Pray, Love* by Elizabeth Gilbert—a book I thoroughly enjoyed. There is something really special about giving yourself an opportunity to explore who you really are. I believed that before I had cancer, and I feel it even stronger now that I've had cancer, not once but twice.

We only have this one life.

This one life.

And it is short and long and terrible and wonderful—my *P.S. I Love You* reference because it's one of my very favorite movies. I can go on and on about why. But that's for another time.

Now to throw the book and movie together—see how my mind works? LOL!—we only have this one life like the movie says, and I see many people slug through it every day with blinders on. So, to see someone really want to connect with who they are, as in the book, is beautiful.

Which brings me to pity and fear.

During the first round with cancer, I was terrified. Losing my mom at such a young age combined with the circumstances at home had a profound effect on making my biggest fear now my kids losing me.

But I felt stronger during the first treatment cycle—which is weird because I've heard most people feel stronger during a second diagnosis since they've already done it and survived once before.

However, I felt as though I had no control, no matter what I did.

I felt hunted.

I'd had a double mastectomy. There was no tissue for the cancer to come back in! I took the proper medication without fail. It should have done its job, especially with all the side effects—at least, that's the complaint I gave. I was exercising, watching what I ate, getting enough sleep every night. Doing all the right things.

The fact that it came back anyway, shocking my doctors—remember that my breast cancer specialist was so surprised she presented my case at a conference?—made me feel like the cancer was targeting me specfically.

Suddenly, I was once again faced with the fear and the appointments, surgery and a new medication. I didn't know how I'd feel after losing my ovaries though I secretly was pretty sure I'd feel better. And I had to do it all again, this time with radiation.

I just wanted the shit out of me.

I was angry, and more than once, I wanted to know why the hell it came back.

The proverbial *why me?*

I'd been aggressive with treatment. I believed I'd done everything right. Hell, I'm the one who found my cancer both times. The stupid fucking shit has been in my life from my very first memory.

What. The. Fuck.

Needless to say, this one hit me a bit harder emotionally, and I really counted on Brian to pull me out of my little and big dips in positivity.

All cards on the table, I could be the poster child for a good ugly cry.

As you deal with cancer, know that there will be days you feel really strong. Take a moment to experience and truly be aware of how that feels. Know that on days where that strength seems to be hiding, you will get it back. Our emotions run on a cycle, and you'll have highs, and you'll have lows. But those lows will pass, and you'll find an upswing again.

One thing I recommend is to have someone in addition to your caregiver, whether that's your spouse, best friend, parent, whoever, whom you can rely on and vent to.

Being a caretaker can honestly be quite burdensome and overwhelming, and your main person will want to be there for you every step of the way. That constant support is an amazing, wonderful, generous gift. But as the person going through the illness, we can't shun all other responsibilities and only think about ourselves—we have to consider our caregivers and loved ones, too. Their health and well-being are important. They are living with cancer, too.

Having another person you can cry with and ramble with and vent to and distract yourself with alleviates some of the constant pressure your caregiver may be feeling and offers you a different perspective for conversations and emotions. This will give you another outlet to get things off your chest and out of your body without completely exhausting your partner in life.

This way, every time you do go to them, they can be strong for you. Positive.

And on those days you are not feeling quite so positive, when you're feeling sorry for yourself, angry or frustrated about your circumstances, acknowledge those feelings because they are real. If you pretend they're not there, deep down in your heart and mind, you'll call yourself a liar, and your positivity won't be as effective.

Accept your emotions, whatever they are, and understand that there is a reason you are feeling that way. And *then*, make yourself start thinking about everything positive in your life, and head toward that upswing.

Negativity welcomes you with strong, persistent arms and says, "You belong with me, babe." It's intriguing or mysterious or even comforting, but it's also a trick because underneath the pull of negativity is a jackass who kicks puppies.

Acknowledge your pain and fear, and then come up with coping skills for yourself to head them off. Think of a list of things to be grateful for or solutions that help you feel empowered ahead of time to help pull you through the tough bouts.

I use thoughts of my children all the time. They are thriving and happy and my greatest gift, and their existence and happiness has been a huge motivation for me to find a way to deal with this in a positive, strong manner.

I am a role model for them. I know they look up to me, and I know that they see me much greater than I really am. Part of my job as a parent is to teach them how to manage hard times.

We can't get through hard times if we let our fear and negativity shackle us to a dirty, piss-soaked floor.

It is much easier to face obstacles if you have an idea ahead of time of how you will get around them.

And hugs. Lots of hugs.

I'm not kidding—look up "health hugs" and you will see the science that backs a twenty-second hug.

Get as many as you can, and give as many as you can.

Then, step forward.

CHAPTER NINETEEN

Radiation Can Suck It

The second time around, I had to have radiation on my left breast.

I count myself lucky because I dodged chemo...again.

I'll take that as a win!

The consultation with my radiologist was hilarious.

I called him Dr. Dan because his last name was difficult to pronounce and therefore difficult to remember with my medicated, foggy brain.

Dr. Dan was a young radiologist, and I loved that he really listened to me—he paid attention to my questions, concerns, and opinions.

This is important later.

During my consultation, Dr. Dan went through all the possible side effects and damages most likely to occur as a result of the radiation. Though they target the radiation very specifically, there are certain parts of your body that will still receive a flash of radiation, kind of like the little bit of light that radiates out past the main beam of a flashlight.

They do their best to minimize that flash, but a little bit would hit my heart and my lungs. From what I understand, radiation damage accumulates or worsens over time, so though no issues are visible right now, twenty years down the road when I get a scan, it may show some damage to either my heart or my lungs.

Because of this possibility of long-term issues, it's important that I maintain a heart-healthy diet and exercise to mitigate that damage. Additionally, having my ovaries removed increases my chance of heart problems due to lack of estrogen.

Double whammy to the heart.

And then he went on to talk about other side effects such as fatigue and skin irritation. In other words, my skin might get a little toasty. It's different for everyone.

After all of this, I asked him why people choose radiation if it has all of these negative effects? He wanted to reassure me. "No, no, you definitely want to do it because it is the best bet of killing any breast tissue cells or cancer cells or hibernating bears, whatever you want to call them."

And then he caveated it by saying, "But just so you know, there is no guarantee."

I laughed...like a full-belly, teary-eyes kind of laugh, and the look on his face was priceless.

I put my hand up and said, "You are the worst salesman ever! Basically, all these bad things can and might happen, but it's the best bet for getting any extra cancer cells, but there's no guarantee it'll work. Yes! Sign me up!"

His look was sheepish, but his tone was sincere when he said, "You need to do this. Period."

"I know," I said.

When you go in for your initial appointments, they do all sorts of measuring and adjustments to make sure they are getting the angle just right. And then, at each appointment after, you will be set up in that same exact position.

During this process, if you notice anything different—and I mean *anything* at all in your body that's changed—you must notify your team. A good staff will listen to you.

My second week of treatment, I noticed that when I swallowed, even something as simple as water, it seemed to get caught in my throat and wouldn't move down. It wasn't every time I ate or drank but it was often, and it was unsettling. I looked online and found an association between breast cancer radiation and difficulty swallowing because of a possible flash on the throat.

I mentioned it to the staff, and they said they didn't think that had anything to do with radiation, but when I talked to Dr. Dan, he listened.

Remember that wonderful characteristic of his?

He said, "I've heard of this before. I don't see it often, but let me take a look at your pictures, and we'll make some adjustments."

He looked, he made the adjustments, and within a week, my swallowing issues were resolved.

Don't let the fact that some clinicians may not be familiar with what you are going through stop them from helping you.

You have to be your strongest advocate.

You can be polite but firm and make sure that they are listening.

I will tell you a little bit about one unfortunate radiation visit.

Being under the lens of the radiation machine kind of freaked me out, so I paid very close attention to everything they were doing. If the huge eye of the lens was opened, did it mean my whole body was being radiated? Did it focus when it was closed? Were they taking photos, or did the radiation treatment come through the lens? Since I wasn't clear on any of this, I was a bit paranoid about it.

Ask questions. Instead of remaining paranoid, make them explain it to you.

On this particular day, a different staff member was setting me up. Because I'd had a mastectomy, they wanted the radiation to be in my skin instead of the usual skin-sparing treatment, which directs the radiation to the tissue below. They were targeting any leftover cells beneath that could potentially turn cancerous.

A bolus is a piece of material that directs radiation into the skin. It's moistened and laid over the breast but avoids the axillary area, meaning not in my armpit. Each time a particular clinician was there, she was careful to smooth out any air pockets in the bolus and ensure it didn't reach my armpit, but when she wasn't there, the other team members that applied the material weren't as attentive to those details.

I was doing radiation to make sure the cancer didn't come back. If it wasn't done exactly the same way and as efficiently as the first time, it freaked me out. What if they missed something? Would this all have been for naught?

On this particular day, they were putting the bolus on but had it all up in my armpit with a bunch of air pockets.

They left the room to take pictures and give me the radiation.

And, by the way, when they leave, they close this huge, foot-thick metal door.

Talk about ominous.

They told me it would take a little bit longer because they were both taking pictures and administering radiation, but that was as far as the explanation went. I laid there, stressed out about the bolus and alone as the huge door automatically closed in slow motion.

As they were getting ready in another room, the big lens of the radiation machine was moving all around me in ways I didn't recognize. Usually, metal teeth closed down into a very small, pointed shape for the radiation, but today it opened wide.

And anytime they turned the machine on, the big *BEAM ON* sign on the wall glowed bright red. Bright red to me means *stop* and *alert*!

As they remotely moved the machine around the table where I lay, it hit the molded armrest that ensured I was positioned the same every day and yanked me to the edge.

To say my adrenaline spiked doesn't even begin to describe what was going on inside of me.

I finally hit my limit, and to be honest, I should have said something earlier. But I knew that if I move, they have to start over, and other patients were waiting. So I kept trying to ignore my fear that they were over-radiating me and the fear that something was going terribly wrong.

The machine hitting my table surpassed my threshold, and I finally sat up and said, "You guys are scaring me." I was on the verge of tears, rapidly blinking them back, and mortified. I kept telling myself I was fine, but it's goddam radiation, and I didn't feel fine.

I was scared. No one was telling me anything, and I'd had it.

They came in apologizing and explained to me what was happening. When the lens was completely open, they were just taking pictures, but the same beam illuminates whether it's radiation or just the camera. It would have been nice to know that beforehand.

I explained that this might be good information to share with their patients. I paid close attention to everything they'd been doing, so when it was different from what I expected, it terrified me.

I let them know that going forward, they needed to talk me through the process anytime something was different. "Don't leave me lying here in silence with this big huge machine, wondering if everything is okay. Explain it to me."

Afterward, I went out to my car and buckled up but didn't start my car. I sat there, staring out the window.

Then I cried. Hard. I found the entire situation traumatizing. I'd felt out of control and in danger, and it brought up all sorts of shit I hadn't anticipated that day.

I called Brian, and as soon as I heard the soft, comforting rumble of his voice, I cried even harder. In that moment, all I wanted was him.

I'm telling you this not because things like this happen often, and even this situation was an anomaly for this radiation clinic—they're quite wonderful, actually.

But when something goes awry—and something will— you need to have a person who will help hold you up until you're ready to stand on your own two feet again.

It'll often only take seconds, but what a difference it makes to have someone to go to. Have that someone set up ahead of time. Don't wait until you need a steady hand to start looking for one. Have it—have them—on the ready.

The other reason I'm telling you this is because you always have to be your greatest advocate.

Always.

Too many times, we sit back and tell ourselves that the doctor is the expert and therefore knows what's best, but doctors are also human. Pay attention to what they say and how they say things should be. Pay attention to what's going on in your body and what's normal for you, and say something when it's not right.

Say something when it's different.

Say something when you have questions because you are worth whatever inconvenience that question could possibly bring.

Back to the radiation process.

Some people have skin that handles radiation just fine. Actually, if they've had a lumpectomy instead of a mastectomy, the radiation can be more skin-sparing. But it's different for everyone.

My radiation was all about going after any possible cells that could be lingering along the underside of my skin because all the other tissue in my breast was gone. All I am is implants.

My skin turned red then almost purple, and then it started to slough off, leaving a wet, oozing mess behind. *The pictures are at the end of the book.

The good thing about my mastectomy in this situation was that I lost some sensation, so though the whole area hurt, it didn't hurt nearly as much as it looks like it would. And I'm thankful.

What seemed like the entire top layer of the skin of my left breast sloughed off, including the nipple, which let me tell you is incredibly disconcerting.

During all this time, I was working my day job and writing nights and weekends while my family of four plus our dog were in a two-bedroom apartment, sleeping on mattresses on the floor, until our house was complete. I had my radiation appointments around seven a.m. before my job started, and during much of my workday, I was slathered in Silvadene and gauze pads under my business suits.

I don't know if I was trying to get through radiation while working and moving our family and enrolling our children into new schools or if I was trying to get through working and moving and preparing my family and kids to start new schools while going through radiation.

Radiation will most likely make you tired.

It may not happen immediately, but then the exhaustion sets in and stays for a while. It wasn't the kind of tired where I couldn't function, but I always felt like I could—or wished I could—lay down and go to sleep. It wasn't easy to maintain a normal pace, but it was doable.

Your mindset and how you are going to tackle treatment can greatly affect how easy or hard you find it. And your life situation may complicate things or enable you to sail right through. I hope the latter for you. Because it sucks that you have to go through any of this in the first place.

The last thing I want to let you know is this—if you take a look at the photographs in the back of the book, keep in mind that at all of it heals, and it all gets better. They are not there to scare you but to prepare you. Don't look if that's not how YOU work.

They are there to prepare you for whatever may come. This way, you aren't shocked, you aren't surprised, and you don't think that you're having some rare reaction to radiation.

My pictures present one normal possibility that may occur with radiation. Preparing myself is half the battle, so if you operate in a similar fashion, these pictures are for you. If you find that seeing raw, weeping skin, or knowing something ahead of time makes you more nervous, then skip it.

That's why they're in the back and not within these pages.

All of my skin healed, and it healed very quickly. Other than looking a little bit tan, no one would know that my skin reacted poorly. And don't worry, I put good pictures in the back, too, to ease any concerns about healing you may have.

One phenomenon I have found is that when you're going through something difficult, even if you know it will end, there can sometimes be a small, persistent worry that it may go on forever.

Pictures may help you see that you will get through it, and not only will you be okay, but if you set yourself up right, you will be stronger and better than ever before.

Then, step forward.

CHAPTER TWENTY

Taking Control

This section is a pep talk.

As I've said before all over this book, you must be your biggest advocate. Knowing your body, knowing what is right for you, or being sensitive enough to at least know if something *isn't* right, is hugely important, not only for you physically but also mentally, emotionally, professionally, and spiritually.

Construct a roadmap of where you are and where you need to be. Then list the actions you feel would get you there. You may not yet have all the answers on how to get from point A to point B. That's okay. Write down the names of people you can ask. And if you don't know who to ask about a particular topic, then speak to whichever of your doctors you feel most comfortable with.

Whether it's your oncologist or your radiologist or your chemotherapy nurse or your psychologist if you go to one—I cannot overstate how highly I recommend you do—tell them about your roadmap. Ask them questions, and invite their feedback. Many people don't even realize how much they want to help others until asked. Besides, these are medical professionals—it's kind of in their genes.

Prepare. Get your mind in a good place. A solid plan that keeps you moving forward can help ease fears that crop up. It can help you walk on through.

There are people who swear by second opinions, third opinions, fourth opinions...well, you get the point. I even read one book where the woman had nineteen *second* opinions before she was finally able to move forward with a treatment plan. Each individual has unique needs —though I couldn't wait that long because comfort comes from action for me—but everyone falls onto the research/action spectrum somewhere.

I was afraid of many of the treatment options, like chemotherapy, but I also knew that if my doctors said chemo was my best chance, then I was taking it regardless of the risks.

My number one goal was survival.

To be here for my kids.

They are my motivation every day.

You might have a different goal or motivation. Determine what is right for you and your individual situation.

Just don't be a complacent patient.

If you have questions, if you have ideas, ask and tell someone. And if you ever have a doctor who pushes back or tells you not to question them or acts annoyed when you bring things up, then I strongly recommend that you find a different doctor.

The first time a doctor thinks they know everything is when they start missing things and making mistakes.

I took control when I told the doctor I wanted my ovaries removed instead of taking the Lupron shot to shut them down. I knew that the combination of my history with my hormones, the side effects of trying to block the hormones with Tamoxifen, everything I researched about Lupron, my age, and the length of time I would have been on that shot that removing my ovaries made the most sense.

I'd felt as strongly about that as I had about the mastectomy.

There was no second-guessing or self-doubt.

I wasn't messing around.

I'm not a doctor, but I'm an intelligent woman who knows her body, knows its patterns, and with the information before me, felt strongly about my decision.

So...be strong, be bold, ask, listen, and identify what is right for you.

Then, step forward.

CHAPTER TWENTY-ONE

Bye Bye, Ovaries, Don't Let the Door Hit Your Ass on the Way Out

As I mentioned in the last section, taking control for me was getting rid of my damn ovaries.

My cancer was hormone-positive, and for years, my body had been notorious for making extremely high amounts of estrogen. Anyone with hormone issues knows that the constant flux makes you feel awful —you deal with fatigue, you can't sleep, you have nausea, aching joints, acne, you're fuzzy-headed, nervous, moody...the list goes on and on.

My body needed balance even if that balance was a very low level of hormones.

We scheduled the removal of my ovaries concurrently with the removal of the skin on my breast where the cancer reoccurred. I found this to be a very quick and easy recovery. They did not take my uterus because all the tests showed that it was healthy.

If it's not broke, don't fix it. Ever hear that saying? LOL! It definitely applies to body parts.

I wanted no part of removing it then, later, dealing with a dropped a bladder or other issues. I was two months into my new job at this point, with the warning that I shouldn't let the cancer affect too much of my workday, so I scheduled the surgery for Thursday and planned to return to work the following Wednesday.

I'd hoped that was enough time for me to get back on my feet and do my job.

A few interesting things happened on this journey.

When you have laparoscopic surgery in your abdomen, they use air to create space. But if all of that air doesn't come back out, it can move around and lodge against nerves.

Whoa.

Let me tell you, the pain can be excruciating.

As Friday wore on, I developed a very sharp pain in my right shoulder. It was a cold and sharp ache, similar to an abscessed tooth. The funny thing about this pain was I knew it wasn't real as far as any actual damage was concerned. In fact, it was radiated pain from my abdomen that had moved up into my shoulder. But the ache was so extreme that it felt almost impossible to pull in any air, making it incredibly hard to breathe. Changing positions did not help ease the pain, and I couldn't tolerate lying down at all. I writhed all over the couch, seeking relief.

My children were nine and eleven at this point, and I hated scaring them, but I couldn't help myself. We reassured them that I wasn't in any danger and nothing was actually injured. I just had to wait for the symptoms to subside, and we were going to go to the emergency room to help manage the pain.

We tried to use it as a learning opportunity to show how, when things are in a heightened emotional state, you can stay calm, ask questions, and make a plan. Brian called the OBGYN doctor who performed the surgery and took me to the emergency room.

They did a few tests to make sure there was nothing serious happening, like an embolism, then gave me morphine. After what seemed an eternity, the pain began to fade. Staying in an upright position kept me most comfortable, but lying down made the air bubble press on that nerve and brought all the pain back.

When we got home, I sat straight up for a little bit even as the pain returned. I joined Brian and kids in the apartment building's activity room and paced in circles while they played pool. Standing and walking felt way better than sitting or lying down, but I was exhausted.

By 11 p.m., I wasn't sure when or how I was going to be able to go to sleep. We were still sleeping on mattresses on the floor, so I finally stacked a bunch of pillows against the wall and slept upright. Not the most comfortable night, but it worked in a pinch.

If you are ever in this situation, a lounge chair with a footrest might be your best bet to comfortably sleep upright.

This does not happen to everyone, and it isn't always quite as bad, but know that this *can* happen. Knowledge keeps you from panicking.

I have spoken to so many people who have had the same procedure done with no issue whatsoever. I guess I'm just lucky! LOL!

Overall, I really do feel fortunate. As I recovered from ovary removal, I started to feel better than I have in years.

The first few weeks, your abdominal muscles are sore, and you're tired because surgery takes a heavy toll on the body. Your whole system is in flux. There's a lot of inflammation, and even though it may not look like anything is happening, your body is working day and night to heal.

That kind of work is exhausting.

Be gentle with yourself.

Healing is not always a standard process, so it may take days, weeks, or months after a procedure for you to feel normal again. Your body will take the time it needs to fully recover—don't rush it, and also don't use this as an excuse not to live.

As I mentioned, I feel lucky because after a few weeks, my body found a balance that it hadn't experienced in a long time. Outside of a few hot flashes, I started sleeping better. I had more energy. All the water I'd retained on Tamoxifen was gone. And my overall feeling of well-being greatly increased.

For a little while.

But hormones take a while to balance, and every shift can cause new symptoms. Lacking estrogen may eliminate—even if only temporary—a few things you hadn't expected or don't notice right away.

I'll get into this more later.

I hope and pray and fervently send out positive vibes that you find your place of well-being.

Another potentially fraught situation I hadn't counted on was my first visit back to see my OBGYN.

After my surgery, I found myself sitting in the office for a follow-up. There I was, forty-two years old, post-menopausal, and in a room full of pregnant women—some of whom were not too far from my age.

I am giving you a head's up about this because, depending on where you are in life, what *your* story is, this can affect you differently. I was fine. It was just something I noticed, and I found it intriguing. I'd already had the children I wanted, and I had no desire for any more, so there was no sadness or sense of loss. It was simply an interesting awareness that I was now in a different state of being than I had been in a very significant way.

Boom. Just like that. I could no longer have children.

Weird but okay.

Some of you may have a different story. Your illness may have affected your ability to have children, and for that I'm so truly sorry. If this situation would be difficult for you emotionally, talk about it with the office so you can wait in a different room, or find a way to address it before finding yourself surrounded by pregnant women. And please, have someone go with you. Someone who keeps you distracted and at ease.

Sign up for a survivor group, or schedule an appointment with an oncology therapist.

Another aspect I hadn't considered... My daughter and I were hanging out together and casually talking about my surgery. She suddenly stopped what she was doing and slowly turned her head toward me with a look of disbelief and a little bit of accusation on her face. Definitely disappointment.

"Wait a minute," she said. "Does this mean you won't have your period anymore?"

Before I caught on to the issue, I threw my fist up in the air and said, "You got it! I'm free!" And I started to laugh.

Thank goodness my kid is so lighthearted. She hid her face with her hands in mock despair and said, "No! Now I'm all alone. I thought we'd be period buddies."

That sobered me up very quickly, and a nudge of what could never be tried to settle in.

For a second, it took away a little bit of the bonding experience I always knew we'd have, dealing with our cycle together. But I also knew that I could still have that with my daughter because I had gone through everything she would be going through, and I could empathize.

And truth be told, I'd already been getting jerked around by her cycle changing mine. I definitely did not have the alpha vagina in our house!

In the end, it was a relief, not having to deal with it anymore.

I assured her I would still be there for her every step of the way, and also, how lucky was I (with appropriate good-hearted taunts and snickers)?

Over the last few years, I started to have really bad pain during ovulation. I had cysts that would grow and then burst after a few days. When the cysts were large, they took up space and caused a lot of pain. I'd have three days when sitting, walking, and sex were painful because anything that pushed against that area made it feel like it was severely bruised.

As soon as they take took my ovaries, I never had pain mid-month again.

At this point, I was thrilled they were gone. Arrivederci, ovaries!

I appreciate the gifts you gave me, but we're done here.

Despite all the "good" things that came from removing my ovaries, other problems snuck up on me and placed me solidly into a heavy state of denial.

Looking back, I can clearly see what had happened, but in the moment, I was too scared and too pissed to admit it...

My sex drive had plummeted.

The connection and intimacy that Brian and I formed in moments together has always been very important to us. The idea that my body wasn't responding, wasn't recognizable literally or figuratively, terrified me into shutting out reality.

I was making sure we had sex around once a week, which was less often than before my diagnosis, but I wasn't making sure we were connecting. With everything going on in our lives, I was exhausted, stressed, and now scared shitless that I was forty-two years old and all my sexy was gone.

My body felt and looked unrecognizable. I didn't feel the way I used to. My body acted like it didn't understand pleasure.

It was a stranger to me.

When Brian would try to talk to me about it, I'd resist out of humiliation and fear. I'd argue back in complete denial. I was so worried my sex drive wouldn't come back, knowing that could ruin our relationship, that I couldn't even admit it to myself, much less him.

And that caused a lot of pain.

Since I didn't explain to him why I hurried through sex now, tried to get through it quickly, remained disconnected, it left him feeling that I didn't want him, didn't find him attractive, or possibly even didn't love him.

I didn't explain any of these things because, honestly at the time, I couldn't accept that it was even happening.

Remember when I said I should have been going to support groups or a therapist to make sure I had help navigating a new normal?

Yeah...this was a big one. I should have been going. They could have helped me understand that there was a very real chance my body would adjust and all my sexy would come back.

Instead, I'd roll over in my misery while my poor husband rolled over in his, thinking it was him I was turning away from, when the truth was that I was turning away from the unrecognizable lump that was my body from my neck down.

When I finally realized how truly rejected my actions made him feel, I was horrified because I love this man with my every breath. It was my intense fear of losing him in the first place that blocked me from communicating and, in the end, put my marriage at risk.

It took almost a year and a half, but my body finally did adjust, and all those stirrings and desires and wants came crashing back.

I wanted to shout hallelujah, but I had a marriage with a lot of pain and anger to work to heal.

As you go through these treatments, remember that our bodies are intricate machines where subtle changes can trigger huge shifts. Give yourself time. Have patience. Stay aware.

Communicate! Let your loved one know how you feel, and get help in understanding what is happening to you physically and emotionally so you don't do what I did.

Don't hurt yourself in that way—my fear and devastation in thinking that part of my life was ruined was excruciating...and it didn't have to be.

Don't hurt someone else.

Go to a support group, a therapist. Research symptoms and side effects. Know what to expect, and learn how to manage it all. Be prepared and ready ahead of time.

Then, step forward.

CHAPTER TWENTY-TWO

Slow and Steady

I was very fortunate to receive the "you're cancer-free" announcement a second time.

Just like the first time, it was accepted with relief and trepidation. Gratitude and fear. I'm so glad it's all gone, but you may find that any time a cough lingers too long, or you have a bad headache, or your hip begins to ache that your first thought will be, "Fuck, it's cancer."

But you will get through this. You will acknowledge that fear and then put everything you know about your current situation into perspective. Including the fact that as we get older, aches and pains, floaters in your vision, lingering coughs after a bad cold can all be part of the aging process.

If, however, you need reassurance or there is something telling you that whatever is going on needs to be checked, call your doctor. Don't mess around. Don't wait. Just go, and put your mind at ease. That way, if it *is* something, you are hitting it fast and furious. And if it is nothing, which often times will be the case, you can rest easy instead of having the fear hover in the back of your brain.

I was cancer-free, and I finished my radiation. I was still more than thirty pounds overweight from the first round of treatments, I was tired, and I felt a bit disconnected—part of losing my ovaries and the body adjustments that come after.

And I had a moment of disgust about the entire situation because, damn it, the person I saw in the mirror was not me.

Truth be told, this type of moment happened often, and it is one of the reasons behind this book. It is one of the very hard lessons I'm trying to teach myself.

I was so impacted by how I felt and how I looked that I disregarded the very real strength it took for me to get through everything I had so far.

Yes, I had amazing support. My husband and children were my very own superheroes.

Regardless, I know it took a survivor mindset from my own perspective.

That's something I've had my whole life and something I hope you have also or that you can develop.

When faced with a problem, I like to come up with a plan that is broken into steps so that I can tackle it methodically. Breaking it into smaller chunks works for me because I can take immediate action—it eases my soul to know that something is being done.

No matter what kind of cancer you have or had—or illness in general—no matter what kind of treatment you faced and pushed through or still remain on, all of this is very hard on your body. It is difficult to wrap your mind around just how strenuous this is for your physical being when you otherwise look fine, but at a cellular and molecular level, there is a battlefield of damage that your body now has to heal and clean up.

This takes time.

Know that whatever nutritional regimen you begin or exercise routine that you start or natural oils, meditation, counseling—this is a must—you pursue, change takes time. The worst thing you can do is try to rush the healing process. You'll only end up more stressed out by setting unrealistic expectations for yourself.

One of the things you have to realize is that your body is different. Your metabolism, the way it functions, has been altered from how it used to work. Expecting the same thing out of it is an exercise in futility.

Acknowledge that in a way, you were a victim. Then, release it.

Do not stay in a victim mentality. It serves no one.

No one.

And least of all, you.

You can look at studies upon studies about survivors, and one of the patterns or common threads is a survivor mindset. You might be facing shit. You might be going through a very difficult time. It might be terrifying and hard and awful, but a survivor mindset will acknowledge that and then say, "Damn it, I am not going to just sit here and let this happen. I am going to actively move through this to my place of health and well-being."

For yourself and for those who love you and for those you love.

As a woman, I faced some pretty major body image issues throughout all of this—I also know this triggered old childhood issues of self-worth I'd never worked through.

I was thirty pounds heavier, and it was all in my belly and hips as you can see on the cover, settling there in the form of cellulite. I had never even known you could have cellulite on your stomach! For someone who had always worked out and watched my nutrition, it was a huge blow. Not to mention the trauma and changes to my body from the mastectomy and the reconstruction and multiple surgeries.

All of those hardships had to be worked through. All of your issues will need to be worked through.

I caution against just accepting less than what you want.

I caution against not working on your emotional well-being as hard as you work on your physical well-being.

There was no way in hell I was going to let this take any more away from me, including my self-esteem and comfort with myself.

In the past, I had tried everything to lose the Tamoxifen weight— intermittent fasting, Keto, calorie counting, and so much more. But no matter how diligently I stuck to my plans, I could not lose any of the weight or burn any of the fat or even gain muscle.

It drove me insane.

It was very demoralizing.

But I kept at it because I knew working out helped me not continue to gain, and it improved my cardiovascular health.

Working out so hard also helped me maintain the muscle mass I already had, which would benefit me in the future. During exercise, my body fueled itself by turning my muscle into glycogen and burning that rather than fat. So no muscle gain, no fat loss, but also, no muscle loss. All very frustrating even as I tried to keep that silver lining in mind.

At this point, my ovaries were gone, my radiation was done, and I was on a new medicine called Aromasin that blocked any extra estrogen made by my lovely abdominal fat and adrenal glands.

And I had a body I didn't like.

If you find yourself in this situation, look in the mirror and truly appreciate and celebrate how amazing and strong your body is for making it through your diagnosis and treatment journey.

Because it is the truth!

But I also know that how we feel about the fact that our appearance affects how we feel about ourselves. As much as we don't want to be controlled by our outside self, we often struggle with its power over our internal worth.

The Look Good Feel Better Foundation is a place you can turn to.

They are online and easy to access with a plethora of tools to help you find little ways to take care of yourself and feel better.

They offer tips about skin care, makeup, hair styles, and even how to style your hair as it comes back in after chemotherapy. There are so many ways to give yourself some TLC and regain confidence.

If brushing your teeth and adding a little lip balm makes you "presentable," consider how learning new makeup applications to enhance your beautiful eyes or discovering new clothing styles that flatter your curves might make you feel.

Throughout my process, I looked for ways to find my way back to me. To my new sexy—whatever that was going to be. Heart-healthy nutrition was part of my care regimen as well.

I called my long-time friend, Amy, who is also a dietician. I caught her up on all of my discoveries. Then, we discussed my need for a nutritional plan that would help me lose weight and protect my heart. She sent me information from the Cleveland Clinic about the protein-sparing modified fast (PSMF).

Cleveland Clinic has a wonderful program that includes Skype sessions with a counselor for accountability and tracking. This is a strict nutritional plan and requires periodic health check-ups to ensure you're maintaining proper vitamin and nutrient levels. If you ever follow this or any other nutritional plan, do it right. Always check with your physician before starting any new nutritional plan to make sure it is healthy for you and your circumstances.

Our bodies are so individual that what works for me may be harmful for you, and vice versa.

One of the things you have to watch for while on PMSF is low levels of potassium. Thanks to my hormones—note: sarcasm—and no estrogen, my testosterone started acting up, and I had bad acne on my chin. My doctor put me on Spironolactone, an androgen blocker which stops the testosterone from having such a strong effect.

Spironolactone also happens to keep potassium in your body.

These two elements were a good balance for my plan.

When I discussed this with my oncologist, he agreed that PSMF could be a good fit for me and that he would help monitor my potassium levels. Spironolactone can also decrease sex drive. So, considering my earlier situation, I needed to be careful of that.

It wasn't easy, but I set myself up for success by making sure that I had the food I could eat around me at all times. Then I found a few ways to carry me through. For example, people who are following the diet only for weight loss are told not to drink alcohol. My biggest concern was keeping my sugars low, and I wasn't worried about small amounts of alcohol slowing down my fat burning. So I would pour myself a tiny bit of ice-cold Prosecco and sip on it in the evening to avoid breaking down and eating sweets or snacking. Find the little tricks that work for you.

My husband takes a few mouthfuls of canned whipped cream. Just enough to ease his sweet tooth in the evening but not enough to add too much sugar.

Little-by-little, I dropped the weight, and now I'm back to my pre-cancer weight. I've slowly figured out how to add exercise back into my daily life. I learned that reasonable goals make success much easier to achieve. For example, my commute and schedule don't allow for an hour at the gym every day, so I try for thirty minutes. That half hour could be an online yoga class or a jog outside or utilizing the gym in my community versus driving to the big gym that's fifteen minutes away.

What I can fit in may not always be my ideal workout situation, but it is a healthy and positive modification to make sure that I am exercising. And in the end, not being ideal is only an excuse we use to avoid life in general...don't do it with your health.

So, stop that.

Start now, not on Monday.

Set manageable expectations.

Small steps.

We have to be careful with perfectionism.

If we have it in our mind that unless we can do this one thing this one way, we won't do it at all, then we're not going to get anywhere. Success is not binary—it's not all or nothing.

Oftentimes, good enough is exactly that. Good enough. Meeting seventy percent of a goal is much better than meeting zero percent.

It is value added and a good decision toward a healthier lifestyle since that's what we're talking about here.

I've also learned that meditation and deep breathing for relaxation are extremely important. I know some people may laugh and scoff at it, but there's no denying the many benefits to your health—mental and physical.

Things don't have to be difficult to be effective. At the same time, things that seem simple may be extremely difficult, but that doesn't mean you should back away from them.

Meditate. Find a moment to sit with your thoughts. Thoughts that are raging at you about the decisions you made, where you are in life, the weight you gained, the things you've missed out on, can be very emotional and exhausting. If we can acknowledge those thoughts and then change our mindset to think about what we are grateful for, what things in our life we do love, those positive thoughts of gratitude will make a changes at a chemical level in your brain that is very real.

Healing is not fast; changing your body and your emotional state is not quick. But slow and steady will definitely win the race.

We don't get anywhere by not doing anything. It seems so simple, but how many of us just don't try at all if it seems hard? How many of us put the things we want in life on perpetual hold? Start with small steps, one at a time, and they will accumulate until, before you know it, you've achieved *something*.

Motivation starts the process but commitment makes us successful.

These goals will be more achievable if we break them down into smaller, more manageable goals so that we are giving ourselves constant positive feedback that we are progressing. This will keep you moving in the right direction.

You've got this. And if you are aren't sure, email me. I'll talk you through it.

Then, step forward.

CHAPTER TWENTY-THREE

The Easy Cancer Killed My Mom

There is an infuriating assumption that I have come across as a breast cancer survivor.

I've been told by a few different people, "You're lucky, you had the *easy* cancer."

I count my blessings every day. I am grateful to be well. I am grateful that I wasn't so sick that I wasn't able to recover.

But those words bewilder me.

At this point, I've had my breasts removed, my ovaries removed, more cancer removed, three additional reconstruction surgeries, and have been on several medications with not-so-fun side effects. I have another surgery scheduled in September. I feel much better now, and yes, I believe I'm going to be fine. But getting to this point hasn't been easy.

And it certainly wasn't easy for my kids or husband or brothers or friends.

The word *easy* is dismissive. It undermines my fear and that of my family.

In fact, I even tried to brush off the seriousness of the situation. But Brian nipped that one in the bud immediately. After my first round with breast cancer, once I was free and clear on the other side, I said, "It's all like it never happened. I'm fine."

He let me know right away that he wasn't okay with that take after what we had gone through. "No, you don't get to do that. The threat was real. Our fear was real. You *are* fine, but that's only because you went at this hard."

I've been told my cancer was *easy* because I had hormone-positive invasive ductal carcinoma, and I didn't have to do chemotherapy. Hormone-positive breast cancer means there are more options for treatment, more chances that something will work. Which *is* a huge blessing.

But I eluded chemo only because I found it early and because I chose a double mastectomy as the initial treatment plan. Had I chosen a lumpectomy, then I would have done both chemo and radiation as well as Tamoxifen. I made the choice to lose my breasts to save myself from chemo.

I did the mastectomy. I went on Tamoxifen.

And guess what? It still came back.

I felt like nothing could keep it away. I dodged chemo the second time because, again, I caught it before it spread. That time, they took my ovaries, cut out the reoccurrence, and put me on Aromasin.

I am so grateful I didn't have to do chemo. I've seen the painful effects it had on my mother, on many friends. But there is also a lasting effect that comes with having a mastectomy, going through a reoccurrence, plus all the fear and uncertainty.

Having to tell our children.

But the biggest emotional gut punch to being told I had the *easy* cancer?

The *easy* cancer killed my mom when I was seven.

There wasn't anything *easy* about that at all.

So please, let's choose our words carefully. Let's be sensitive to each other's challenges even if we think our own are harder.

There is nothing *easy* about any of it. Every one of us has our own journey to face, and in each moment, the fear and pain and discomfort are as real as anyone else's.

All of it is hard.

But hopefully, we are surrounded by loved ones to help us through.

Was I lucky? Fortunate? Blessed? Hell, yes. I am all of those things.

And beyond grateful.

There are diseases out there that don't allow for a happy ending. But so far, I'm trying to have mine.

Tell a hormone-positive breast cancer patient she may be fortunate, but don't tell her she had it *easy*.

Or, if you've been told the same, take a deep breath, and let it all roll away.

Then, step forward.

CHAPTER TWENTY-FOUR

But You're So Pretty
and Good Intentions that Hurt

People generally want to relate and connect with one another.

When we meet someone new, we tend to look for commonalities, something that will connect us, but all of us aren't always good at it.

Through diagnosis or treatment or healing and finding your new normal, you may encounter people who say upsetting things. I want you to be ready with a thoughtful phrase of comfort for yourself, so that if it happens, you can let it pass and not allow it to ingrain itself into your day or your heart.

These are all true stories.

One afternoon, I had time between client appointments and work meetings, so I popped into a cancer support organization to learn about some of the support programs they had—the classes and workshops, group meetings, and any events that were coming up. I hadn't attended any of these classes but circled around and considered it every now and again.

I'm telling you—now, again—to go. Don't just consider it. I recommend them for you, because even though each of us is different, sometimes having other people to talk to who are going through the same thing makes a huge difference. I'm a writer, and talking to other writers about the challenges has a certain satisfaction to it that I don't get by talking to people who don't write. Same for dealing with and getting through trauma.

As I was speaking with a woman about the cancer support programs, she gave me an odd look and said, "Do you know someone who had or has cancer?"

"Me. I'm a two-time breast cancer survivor." I was dressed in a business suit and didn't "look" sick, so I assume she thought I couldn't be there for myself.

The woman's eyes went wide, and she was slack-jawed for a second before she said, "But you're so pretty."

Her words left me numb. Hollow.

I can't tell you how long I stood there, blinking at her in surprise.

It felt like ages, but I'm sure it was a blip.

And then she caught herself and put her hand over her mouth. "I didn't mean to say that. I know that cancer is not prejudiced."

I know she was just giving me a very nice compliment regarding my appearance, but I was shocked by two things. Number one, the notion that bad things don't happen to attractive people and their lives are easy; and number two, the idea that if someone is *un*attractive, then they are somehow more deserving of bad things.

Neither of these things is true.

Facebook is populated with well-intentioned people. I'm a romance author and have a loving and supportive writing community. From day one of my diagnosis, I've been an open book, sharing the journey and all my feelings about love.

Doing so opens me up to other people's opinions, some of which are extremely helpful and others, not so much.

During my first diagnosis, I can't tell you how many people responded with loving kindness but added in the same comment that a family member or friend had died from the same thing.

It's always jarring to read.

I took the stories as they were meant—to connect and offer love. I tried not to think about the oblivious negativity that was shared. It may not have affected me as much at first because my mother had also passed from breast cancer, and I knew what I was fighting.

Within minutes of announcing that my cancer came back during the second diagnosis, I received two Facebook messages from real-life friends, not FB acquaintances, who told me that they had a close family member or friend whose cancer came back the second time, and they died.

I know that they were simply trying to connect with me. I know that these two people love me and never, in any way, intended to scare me more. But with the second diagnosis, I went through a weird time where I felt a bit hunted. I worried when my husband and children were away from me. I worried getting on elevators. I worried if I had to travel...as if the universe was out to get me.

Hearing those two stories shook me more than anything else during this journey. I was in my bedroom, my heart was pounding, and I was shaking and crying. I went looking for Brian because he's my person. He was sitting on our living room ottoman, playing a video game, and I dropped to my knees in front of him and threw my arms around his midsection, crying and saying, "I don't want to die."

He held me and reassured me.

I calmed down and put it all into perspective.

I'm sharing this with you so that if anyone says something that seems insensitive, try to keep their intent in mind. Sometimes, the most well-meaning of us make mistakes in how we're trying to connect.

Find your person to help you through it.

Then, step forward.

CHAPTER TWENTY-FIVE

I AM ME

Talk about wonky.

That surgery for September that I mentioned earlier was supposed to fix the very wonky breasts you see on the front cover. My left side reacted to the radiation with an encapsulation—scar tissue formed around the pocket of my implant and got really hard.

My breast tissue was literally as solid as an apple.

My amazing plastic surgeon, Dr. Wendy, tried to lift the other breast to gain some symmetry. And though her work on the right breast was beautiful, there was no way to lift it high enough. Even if there had been, the encapsulated one kept rising and moving toward the center.

We were going to give it one more try the following April, but she recommended me to one of her colleagues, Dr. Frank, for a DIEP flap surgery. This was the only way to ensure that the encapsulation wouldn't return, because once that scar tissue shows up, it doesn't want to leave. Removing it all together is the only real solution.

A DIEP flap is when they take the skin, fat, and vascularization of another area on your body—mine was my stomach, silver lining!—and use it to rebuild your breast.

The microsurgery required to reattach venous supply is fascinating, and I'm in awe over what our medical community can do.

Dr. Frank was amazing and did a spectacular job. Life changing in a way I'm not sure he'll ever quite fully understand.

I'm forever in Dr. Wendy's debt for referring me out, based on the goals I had for myself.

I will let you know this surgery is big.

And I severely underestimated it. LOL! I wanted to jump back into work in two weeks and be on my way.

The world had other plans, but I did get through it just fine.

I just had to be patient.

So that you, too, can manage expectations, know that you need someone there to care for you. Be patient in your recovery. It will be hard to stand up straight for a while, which makes your back ache, but you will get there.

Patience, gentleness, hope.

All these things will help you through.

I've added one more picture right after this passage.

This is me now.

There is something I hope that you can find within yourself.

And that is LOVE.

You see, the woman on the front cover and the woman you see here have both showed tremendous strength and courage in her life. She's very loving, generous, full of forgiveness. She is flawed, stubborn, and gets a bit too focused at times. She's had trauma and joy, failures and success, great love and terrible heartache.

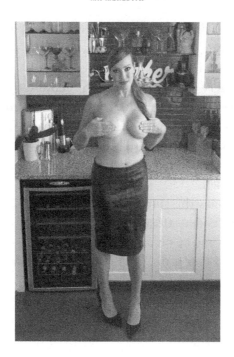

Both women have the same value. Extra weight, scars, wonky breasts...these things do not define us or our value.

We have to learn how to believe that we are more than just this physical shell. We are more than our pain and hurt and fear. We are the all-encompassing sum of echoes that the experiences of our life fill us with.

All of it.

The good and the bad.

We are worthy and valued, no matter if we're wonky or not.

I am me.

And you are you.

Now go ahead...

And take that next step forward.

I'll be here if you need me.

XOXO...

MK Meredith

SYMPTOM MANAGEMENT

These are a few of the symptoms I experienced and options I tried in order to manage them. You may need to try different things until you find what works for you.

*Always speak to your physician about what is right and safe for you specifically.

My suggestions are only that...suggestions. Speak to your doctor first.

Water retention: Lemon water is very helpful when dealing with water retention. Diuretics are also an option, but I did not like how dry they made my mouth. So lemon water was my go-to. A LOT of water with lemon. LOL! Speak with your doctor about options.

Difficulty falling asleep: Magnesium is a calming supplement. I would take this before bed, and coupled with a five-minute deep breathing meditation I have on an app called Beltone, I found it often did the trick.

Acne: Once my ovaries were gone and my estrogen was depleted, the imbalance to my testosterone caused cystic acne to creep back into my life. I found that Spironolactone (an androgen blocker) helped decrease testosterone's ability to have an effect, leaving me with clear skin. You'll have to talk to your doctor and adjust the dosage as necessary. This is a potassium-sparing medication, so you'll need to get your blood checked monthly to make sure your potassium levels are healthy. Again...talk to your doctor.

Achy joints: On both Tamoxifen and Aromasin, I have achy joints, but it was worse with Tamoxifen. Either way, I consistently take glucosamine/chondroitin. It has been a life saver! As long as I take it, my joints feel really good. But if I don't, I notice right away.

Weight gain: I followed a modified version of the Protein-Sparing Modified Fast (PSMF) combined with intermittent fasting. Basically, lean meat, mostly green vegetables, low to no sugar, low dairy, and healthy fats. Some days I'd eat my calories between the hours of noon and eight p.m. If you try this plan, educate yourself, and I recommend following it with medical supervision such as the Cleveland Clinic. Again, consult with your physician.

Foggy-headedness: I started taking DHA to help with this. Either my body adjusted, and the fog eased, or the DHA helped. Either way, it's good for me so I continue to take it.

Overall malaise: Talk to your physician about supplements and minerals that you can be taking to boost immunity and energy levels. Do your research, ask questions, and keep going until you get some answers.

TLC Recommendations: (As you can)

Soaks in Epsom salts, deep breathing and relaxation meditation, regular exercise, some kind of art, and music you love. Find a way to incorporate these things into your life at least once a week if not once a day.

Reducing stress is very important for a healthy immune system.

Go to support groups and/or an oncology therapist!

Now...take that next step.

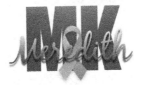

BOOB GALLARY

The following photos will give you an idea of what you can expect with surgery and treatment. Please remember this...it all gets better! These photos are simply to prepare you for what may be and remind you that it will get better. If this works for YOU continue, if not, time to close the book! (to see in color go to mkmeredith.com/not-your-usual-boob/)

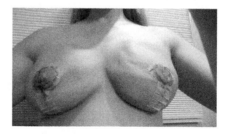

After mastectomy with drains removed. I have tissue expanders in place.

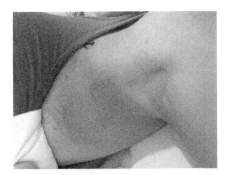

The beginning of my skin reaction to radiation.

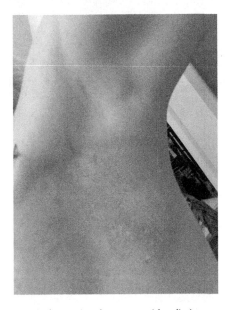

My skin continued to worsen with radiation.

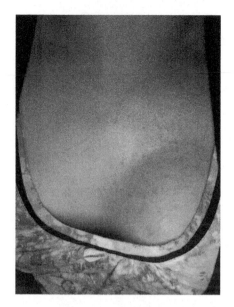

The beginning of my encapsulation from radiation.

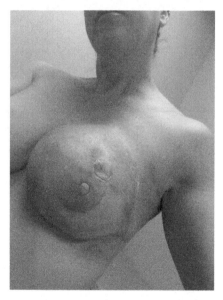

My skin is getting worse, my breast is swollen, and my skin is continuing to deteriorate.

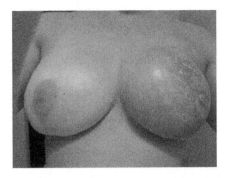

Breast encapsulation is visible, my skin is raw and starting to slough off.

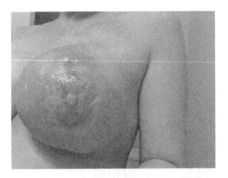

Skin is sloughing off and encapsulation is worsening.

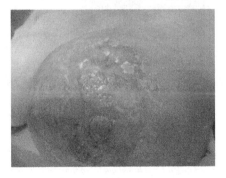

A few days later. Don't worry...this all heals!

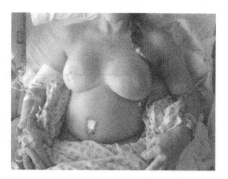

After my DIEP Flap. The breast on the right is very swollen but returns to normal size. This surgery corrected the encapsulation.

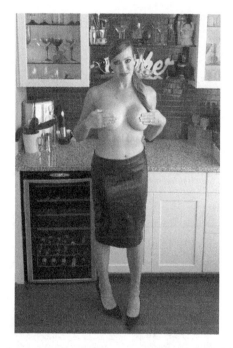

Remember, no matter how bad things seem... with each day, each breath, things will get better. I had this photo taken with my cell phone, a casual remake of the cover, no filters, no special tricks. Just me. Be patient and love yourself. Photo credit: Anya Meredith

ACKNOWLEDGMENTS

Words seem so ineffective when it comes to saying thank you. Especially when dealing with something as difficult as cancer or illness of any kind. I'd been elbows deep in books on cancer that were making me more scared than I already had been when my husband, Brian, suggested I write a book that I'd like to read.

My first thank you goes to him.

Thank you, Brian, for pushing me and loving me through this unwanted invasion. Always remember, you are my favorite.

Thank you to my children for loving me in all my forms while getting these words and emotions on 'paper.'

A huge thank you to Jessica Snyder, not only an amazing friend but a talented editor who gifted the edits of this book to me because she is next-level awesome.

Dawn Yacovetta, I owe you a huge thank you and so much more for being my eagle eyes and pouring over my books.

Lauren Layne! Fellow romance writer and talented designer, this cover...what can I say? Your patience and insight guided us to this beautiful cover. Thank you for taking on this project, and thank you for being so generous and kind. You captured my vision perfectly. Oh! And everyone needs to go read your books!

And to all my fellow breast cancer sisters and brothers and all the caregivers working so hard to help ease the fear and pain...thank you for your grace, strength, and love.

Keep taking that step forward.

ABOUT THE AUTHOR

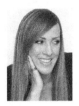

MK Meredith is a two time breast cancer survivor determined to help give comfort to friends far and wide. With a background in occupational therapy, she's gained valuable knowledge in psychology and medicine alike, aiding her own path toward feeling stronger. As a romance author, she pours her heart into as many happy ever afters as she can muster while being thankful for her time with the love of her life and two beautiful children.

I love to connect!
    mkmeredith.com/follow-mk/
    facebook.com/NotYourUsualBoob/

ALSO BY MK MEREDITH

MK Meredith is a romance novelist promising an emotional ride on heated sheets.

Check out her happy ever afters at

www.mkmeredith.com

Cape Van Buren
On the Cape Novels:

Love on the Cape (Larkin and Ryker) bk 1

Honor on the Cape (Blayne and Jamie) bk 2

Cherish on the Cape (Claire and Mitch) bk 3

Draw You In (Sage and Parker)

Scripted for Love Series

There's no place like paradise and the happy ever afters found in the film industry of Malibu, CA.

Love Under the Hot Lights

Just a Little Camera Shy

A Heated Touch of Action

International Temptation Series

A strong dose of decadence along with a side of tall, dark, and sexy in your favorite travel destinations.

Seducing the Tycoon

Playing the Spanish Billionaire

What Happens in Vegas Series

What happens when a romance convention descends upon Vegas? A whole lot of love!

Seducing Seven bk 9

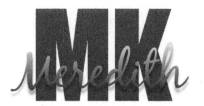